How to stay in love

The happiness for couples workbook

By the same authors:
Love Strategies

How to stay in love

The happiness for couples workbook

**Susan Quilliam and
Ian Grove-Stephensen**

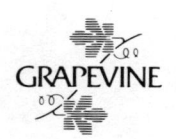

GRAPEVINE

First published 1988
© Transformation Management Ltd.

All rights reserved. No part of this book may be reproduced or utilized in any form or by any means, electronic or mechanical, including photocopying, recording or by any information storage and retrieval system, without permission in writing from the Publisher.

British Library Cataloguing in Publication Data

Grove-Stephenson, Ian
  How to stay in love: the happiness for couples workbook.
  1. Interpersonal relationships. Role of love
  I. Title   II. Quilliam, Susan
  302

ISBN 0-7225-1687-8

Grapevine is an imprint of the
Thorsons Publishing Group,
Wellingborough, Northamptonshire NN8 2RQ

Printed in Great Britain by
The Bath Press, Bath, Avon

10 9 8 7 6 5 4 3 2

Contents

Authors' note	6
Introduction	7
Communication	16
Reading the signs	18
What do you *really* mean?	20
Getting what you both want	22
What might happen?	24
Breaking the news	26
What I really want to say is . . .	28
Environment	30
Ideal environment	32
Creating a home	34
Creating emotional security	36
Personal space	38
Time together, time apart	40
Division of labour	42
Tidiness	44
Other people	46
Family tree	48
Who do we go to for Christmas?	50
Long-term responsibilities	52
Your friends or mine?	54
Work	56
Work and play	58
Working together	60
Money	62
Staying at home	64
Life plan	66
Feelings	68
Self-esteem	70
Individual or partner?	72
Where are you vulnerable?	74
Creative rowing	76
Keeping boredom at bay	78
Jealousy	80
Motivating each other	82
In love forever?	84
Sex	86
Voices from the past	88
First moves	90
There, please	92
Patterns of love-making	94
Open or closed?	96
Contraception	98
Children	100
Shall we have children?	102
What might you feel?	104
Getting support	106
Whose responsibility?	108
Giving the same message	110
Transition points	112
When they've gone	114
Futures	116
The bottom line	118
What if?	120
Growing together	122
Long-term futures	124
Conclusion	126
Resources	128

Authors' note

Like most authors in the 1980s, we have been faced with the quandary of how to express a non-specific gender. The conservative but established 'he' and 'him'? The fashionable but unwieldy 's/he' and 'him/her'? Rigorous alternation of 'him' and 'her', as we used in *Love Strategies*?

We wrote this book for both sexes and it is our hope that it will be read and written in jointly by couples as well as by individuals of both sexes who are interested in the development of sound relationships. However, our publishers tell us from their considerable experience that most people who buy the book will be women. So we have chosen to let 'she' and 'her' stand for the non-specific gender throughout the book.

Acknowledgements

Our thanks to everyone who has made this possible, including all the individuals and couples who gave us the benefit of their experience, especially Maggie Steel for the time and experience she put into helping us prepare the chapter on children.

Introduction

Why a workbook for couples? Surely love is a spontaneous thing, something that happens with the right chemistry, something that doesn't need working at?

Certainly, there can be a magic about love that defies all explanation, that makes your heart beat faster and your knees turn weak, but this magic is not always the stuff that lasting, working relationships are made of. It is the first step, but not the whole journey. When you sort out the idealists from those who are really making their relationships work, then you have people who have struggled, suffered and worked amazingly hard at staying in love.

No lessons in love

The particular problem for people in the second half of the twentieth century is that there are no lessons in love. In our grandparents' time, young people grew up surrounded by couples who were living out the problems and delights of relationship.

As you grew up, you learned what partnerships were all about, from your own parents, your grandparents, the numerous relatives living in the next street or the next room. You lived in very close proximity, but it meant that you learned how successful relationships were run—and how disastrous ones came to be that way.

We don't have all that now. Instead, we have romantic films, idealized novels, and soundproof walls. We never get to know how Mum and Dad make up when they are angry—or make love when they are affectionate. So how are we to learn how to love?

What we need are experiences to help us learn how to structure our relationships, so that we can improve our partnerships and solve our problems when they go wrong. Without making heavy weather of living or loving, we need a workbook for couples.

Who is it for?

How to stay in love is not for those who have perfect relationships, nor for couples who have doomed relationships. If you are in the middle of ending a relationship, this book will not change that, though it may be just what you need next time around.

Equally, it cannot provide an instant 'fix' when a problem rears its ugly head. If you are in the middle of a flaming row, this book will only be useful as a missile! The time to use it is before and after rows, not during them.

If you have a relationship you want to improve, then keep reading. It may be that you are happy, with no immediate dissatisfactions, but simply want to take another step in the deepening of your love. It could be that you know your relationship is basically sound, but you are aware of improvements you would like to make. In particular, if your relationship is in its early stages—if you are engaged, just married, or have just started living together—you may want to lay the foundations of a serious commitment. If you want to stay in love, this book is for you.

You can use this book on your own, although many of the exercises are better done as a couple. You can use it now and again, when an issue occurs, or as a regular part of your communication process. We know one couple who take a regular weekend away, just to revitalize their partnership by looking at it more closely—this book would certainly fit well into their luggage!

What does the book do?

How to stay in love is *not* a textbook; it doesn't contain long passages about the theory of relationships, although it does include some basic ideas about how they work. It is a 'working at' book, not a 'talking about' book. It provides some frameworks or explorations within which you can explore what is happening: you provide the raw material which goes in the frameworks and which makes up your relationship.

Occasionally, the book also gives suggestions as to where to go next, but usually, what you do with the information you gain is up to you. Once you understand your partner, you will know the best way to love him.

This first chapter is a kind of user's guide: it introduces you to the basic ideas behind the book, and then gives you a step-by-step guide on what the book includes and how to use it.

Some basic ideas

There are some basic ideas upon which this book is based, and which you will often find cropping up again. They underpin everything.

- **More knowledge means more success.** The more you learn about each other and about the way your relationship works, the more successful it will be. There is a case for unpredictability in a partnership, and a little bit of uncertainty can often help to keep interest alive, but in general we believe that the more you know about each other, the more you will be able to love each other and stay in love.

- **Everyone is different.** This is self-evident, but often we forget it. It is usually difference that attracts us to each other, and helps us fall in love. When you see someone who has characteristics you like and admire, you are attracted to him—and often these characteristics are ones you want because they are ones you do not have yourself.

- **Difference can create conflict.** As well as creating the excitement that helps us to fall in love, difference can also in time annoy, irritate and destroy. 'If only he did that my way . . .'; 'My wife doesn't understand me', are cries that reflect perennial problems.

- **Difference creates partnerships.** It is this very difference, originally attractive and subsequently irritating, that makes for true compatibility. Because you are different, you can come together to make a fitting, working couple. You can compensate for each other's weaknesses and benefit from each other's strengths. One of the key concepts running throughout this book is that differences, once explored, can be enjoyed as the key factors in true partnership.

How are *you* different?

'Difference' can mean many things. Obviously everyone's different in height, weight, gender, age, and most of us will be aware of basic differences between us in personality. Things that you find funny, leave him cold. She adores sport while you like sitting at home in front of the fire.

If you really want to learn about each other's differences, you can go much deeper than these surface issues. Here are some of the things you can learn about each other at a very deep level. Throughout the book, we will build your awareness of them, and help you find out more.

- **Different pasts create different presents.** Of course, you know that your partner's past is different from yours. You lived hundreds of miles apart as children, you have different careers, but do you know just how he came to be the way he is? Do you know the messages that he carries with him about life, commitment, love, duty? If you can learn these things, through some of the explorations which invite you to identify past messages, you will find it easier to understand your partner.
- **Same word, different meaning.** Even though you use the same words, you may not mean the same thing. How much heartache has been caused through one partner using the word 'love' and meaning 'lust', and the other using the word 'love' and meaning 'commitment'? Quite a number of the explorations in this book encourage you to swap notes about the different ways you use the same words.
- **Different strategies, different strengths.** We each have our own ways of doing things, and, as we said earlier, this may cause irritation but it can also add strength to a partnership. If you can learn more about your partners' strategies—thoughts, feelings, beliefs, ideas and actions—then you will begin to understand why he moves through the world the way he does.
- **Same explicit contract, different implicit contract.** An explicit contract is an agreement you have about some aspect of your lives that you have discussed and come to an arrangement about. Many couples, for example, have explicit agreements about money, fidelity or whether they are to have a family or not. But many of the things you do as a couple are not discussed beforehand. You both *expect* things to be a certain way, you feel you don't need to discuss them; they form your implicit contract. This is fine as long as your expectations are the same. When they are different, you have problems. Resentments build up, disillusionment creeps in—not because you have broken an agreement, but because each of you have unwittingly trampled on expectations that your partner has but you know nothing about. This book will help you to talk about your implicit contracts and realize the differences between them.

How to use the book

The first tip is *don't read it from start to finish*. This is a book to dip into, when the mood strikes, when the need is there. Because of this, it is worthwhile getting to know what the explorations are and what each chapter covers, so that you can find them easily when you want to.

Explorations

The explorations come in a number of forms. What they have in common is that they all gather information, about you, your relationship and, in particular, the differences between you. They also suggest a next step, of exchanging this information and beginning to understand how your differences are useful to you.

There are many different kinds of exploration. Here we give you a 'guided tour' of them.

- *Questions* Explorations usually pose questions about your thoughts, feelings, actions and beliefs. Answer them as honestly and as deeply as you can, without telling things that you would rather not share.
- *Charts* Often explorations are set out in the form of charts or grids to put the information in some sort of order.
- *Gradings* Another way of getting information about issues is to ask you to grade things.

- *Ideals* We often suggest you think of your ideal: ideal home, ideal future, ideal relationship. This is useful because it allows you to think about possibilities you may feel are fantasies. So, for 'ideal' explorations, let your imagination run riot!
- *Brainstorms* If we ask you to 'brainstorm' an issue, this means that any idea about it, however silly, is acceptable. This is a way of allowing you to tap creative possibilities you may have previously discounted.
- *Meanings of words* We sometimes ask you to give your own meanings and equivalents to words, like 'love' or 'fidelity'—to let you compare notes on how your specific ideas of these words differ from your partner's.
- *Speech bubbles* Some explorations invite you to fill in boxes or speech bubbles with what you imagine other people are saying or thinking. This gets you to realize your ideas about them.
- *Completing sentences* Another way of getting in touch with ideas is to complete sentences about them.
- *Pictures* Some of the explorations ask you to draw or fill in pictures, maps or diagrams. This allows you to express your thoughts and feelings in other ways than through words. Don't worry if you can't draw; these explorations are not about artistic talent, but about getting information.
- *Writing space* Some explorations simply give you the opportunity to write down things you may not wish to share face-to-face with your partner.
- *Talking* Obviously! We usually suggest that you discuss together what you've found out from each exploration. Occasionally, we suggest that you structure what you are saying in a particular way, maybe using a form of words that gives information.

How to set up explorations

In the introduction to each exploration, we give you instructions on how to set it up. This will indicate if you need to work alone or together; whether the exploration is best done by writing or talking.

The fact of doing explorations is one that may raise a number of issues for you. Firstly, if only one of you chose to buy this book and the other is not quite so willing to participate, this *does not* mean that your partner is less committed to the relationship than you are. It may only mean that he or she does not want to talk about your partnership in the way this book suggests.

It is possible to learn a great deal about yourself and your relationship by using this book alone. We have usually set up explorations to be done by two of you, but you can interpret our instructions for your own situation.

Secondly, what is the best space, and the best time in which to do the explorations? You will usually need a space that's private, although what you mean by privacy can vary. The safety of your own home may not be private, because of children, pets and open doors. The train to Edinburgh on the other hand, might be an ideal place to do explorations, because it is an anonymous setting with lots of coffee available to help things along!

The amount of time explorations take can vary but they will usually take at least an hour, and you should expect some of them to take longer. Remember that doing the exploration itself may take as little as five minutes, but thinking about what you've both learned may take a year.

It is sometimes possible to do explorations in installments; but make sure you don't underestimate the time an exploration takes, or find yourself in the middle of one when other, more practical matters call!

To help you decide about these issues (and to give you a trial run at doing some), we have two explorations for you to do now. The first is to help you identify just what you hope to gain by using this book.

Exploration 1

Hopes and fears

Think about

You've read about our rationale for writing a couples' workbook—what is your rationale for reading it?

It's useful, before you do anything important, such as taking a job or entering a new relationship, to think about why you are doing it. This will focus your attention, help you get the most out of it, and make you aware of what might go wrong.

The exploration

The drawing gives you several headings surrounding the central issue of this book. Jot down notes as you want to about what your thoughts and feelings are. Don't worry about writing volumes; a few words will do.

If your partner can do the same, so much the better. If not, and you feel that you will probably use this book mostly on your own, it is still a good idea to do this exploration—to remind you of what you as an individual want to give to your relationship.

Afterwards

Once you have written down your thoughts, consider these things, either by yourself or by talking with your partner.

- Are your hopes realistic? Have another look at the book. What will it really give you? What do you yourselves have to input in order to get your hopes fulfilled?

- Are your fears realistic? Will doing the explorations really make these things happen? How could you protect yourselves against them?

- Do your hopes and fears differ from your partner's? Can you reassure each other about fears and enthuse each other about hopes? What is interesting about the difference in your feelings?

- What is the best possible way your relationship could develop through working on it with this book?

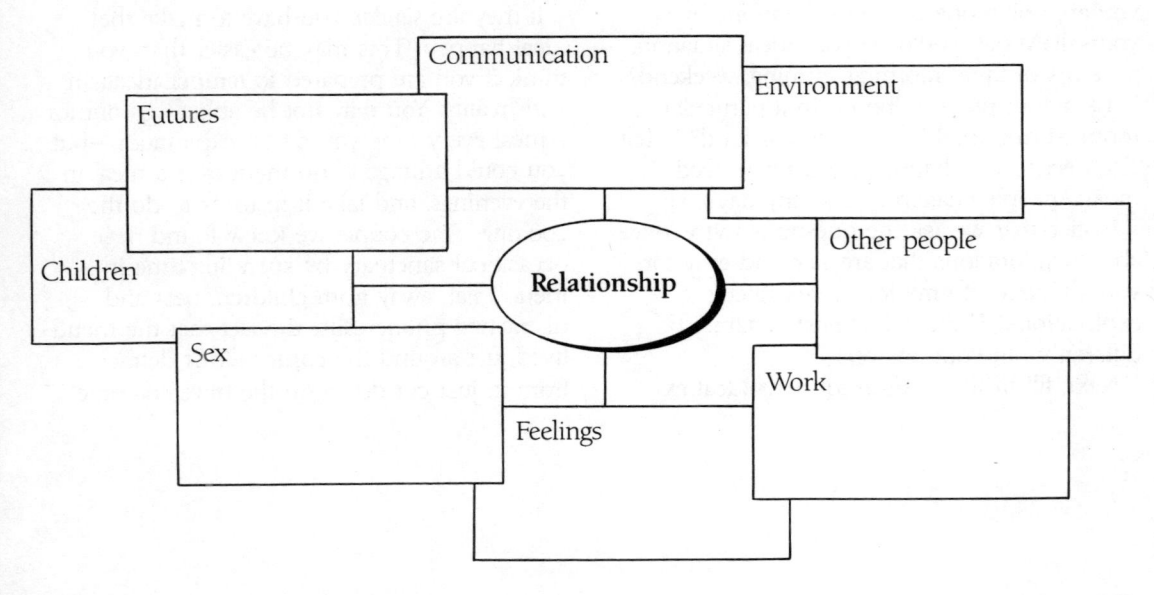

```
         Communication
                              Environment
   Futures
                                        Other people
 Children         Relationship
         Sex                    Work
              Feelings
```

Exploration 2 — When and where

The second exploration is for you to try looking at the practical issues around beginning the explorations.

Think about

Before you begin any of the things we suggest in this book, you need to think about when and where is the best place to do them. First of all, think about your ideal for exploring—what time, what place, what situation?

It could be that you prefer a quiet evening in with a bottle of wine, whereas your partner wants to talk things through over dinner, or in the park. For the moment forget the constraints you have in real life—deadlines, meals to cook, children to collect, and allow yourself to explore possibilities by focusing on your ideal, no holds barred.

The exploration

The grid on the opposite page contains a number of boxes for you to fill in. Imagine you are doing one of the explorations by yourself. What would be your ideal situation, in terms of time: morning, evening, weekend? What about place: at home, in a particular room, surrounded by cushions or food? What else needs to be happening: do you need music, people chattering, a sunny day?

Notice that we ask the questions twice, once about explorations that are safe and easy for you, the second time for more difficult explorations. There will almost certainly be differences in your answers.

Next, fill in the column for your ideal exploration done with your partner. Comment on the same issues—time, space, other things happening.

Then get your partner to fill in the next column about his ideal situation for doing an exploration alone—and then with you. Both of you should write as much as you need—sometimes a few words can be enough.

Afterwards

Once you've filled in the grid, think about your answers and talk them through with your partner, if you can.

The first thing to discuss is whether your ideals of where and when and how are similar or not.

If your ideas of ideal exploration situations are *different*, you have an immediate chance to begin your work on your relationship right now. The fact that you want different things has its good points—begin negotiating what you both need in order to feel happy about doing explorations.

If they are *similar*, you have to make the ideal happen. This may be easier than you think if you are prepared to temper idealism with reality. You may not be able to go out for a meal every time you do an exploration—but you could arrange to do them over a meal in the evenings, and take it in turns to do the cooking. One couple we knew found occasional sanctuary by spending time in a friend's flat, away from children, pets and distracting phone calls: the fact that the friend lived just around the corner didn't detract from it, just cut down on the travelling time!

	You Alone	You Sharing	Him Alone	Him Sharing
Safe Explorations Where do you need to be?				
When is a good time?				
What else needs to be happening?				
Risky Explorations Where do you need to be?				
When is a good time?				
What else needs to be happening?				

Chapter topics

Communication This chapter covers the whole area of communication, one of the key issues for many couples. It can be muddled by fears, misunderstandings and lack of knowledge. It can be too risky even to contemplate. We offer explorations to encourage you to read each other's non-verbal signals more accurately, to understand what you really mean by what you say, and to help you overcome the fear of expressing your real feelings. This chapter also covers negotiating solutions to issues where you both want opposing things.

- **Environment** It may seem as if the environment you live in—your personal space, your home, your neighbourhood—has little relevance to your relationship. Many couples find, however, that creating the right environment supports their partnership. We offer explorations to help you discuss what your ideal environments are, and to plan your home in a harmonious way. We also look at personal space and time, and how differences in your expectations of these can put a strain on your relationship. Finally, we consider how maintaining your environment—by doing housework for example—can be tackled so that you both get what you want.

- **Other people** Whether they are family, friends, or colleagues, other people *do* influence your relationship. They can threaten, support, make or break a partnership—unless you understand what is happening. A variety of explorations look at how you interact with various people in your lives: what expectations your families have of your relationship, and how you can break free of the shackles these impose; how you can meet family needs, in short-term situations, such as visiting for Christmas, and long-term situations such as caring for elderly parents; how you can combine your partnership with your social life—to enhance or conflict.

- **Work** Some couples can keep work and relationships totally separate, whereas others both work and live together. Whichever one is right for you, work (or the lack of it) will impinge on your partnership in a number of ways. Issues concerning money, time, organization and child-rearing all come from the same root—combining work and being half of a couple. This chapter offers explorations about the different values you place on your own and your partner's job, which of you stays at home, how you can work together and who controls the money supply. Finally, a more long-term exploration invites you to examine your work plans and to see how they fit in with those of your partner, and to consider your children's needs.

- **Feelings** Emotions run through every aspect of being part of a couple. However negative feelings can often spoil what is an otherwise healthy relationship. We offer explorations on self-esteem, acheiving a balance between individuality and partnership, and building good feelings for each other. We also look at how to use rows to enhance your relationship, how to motivate your partner and how to stop boredom creeping in. You can use explorations in this chapter to deal with generalized negative feelings, or to tackle a particular set of resentments that is threatening to unbalance your relationship.

- **Sex** One of the elements that can distinguish friendship from intimate partnership is sex. This chapter explores a number of issues about making love. We begin with one to help you identify which past ideas about sex are still useful to you, and which of them you want to let go of so that you can enjoy sex here and now. Three explorations help you communicate what you really want in bed. We then go on to explore what the terms of your sexual contract are; have you agreed monogamy or openness, and is what you agree what you really want? Finally, we look at the responsibilities of making love, with an exploration about finding the sort of contraception that suits both of you.

- **Children** For many couples, the natural development of their relationship is to extend their love to include children. In this chapter, we look at a series of issues where having a family overlaps with being a couple. The first exploration in this chapter provides a structure on which you can base considering the very serious implications of deciding to have children. There are two explorations designed to help you prepare for and cope with being a new parent. They cover emotions, personal limits and your support network. There are then three negotiations on the issues of parental responsibility and the principles you wish to raise your child(ren) by. The final explorations look at what happens when the family leaves home, and you are left alone with your partner.
- **Futures** Building a future together, even if it is only short-term, is a crucial part of any relationship. This chapter looks at different ways of preparing for your future together.

First of all, we look at what would have to happen in order for you to break up, a 'bottom line' that we all need to be aware of, even if only to avoid it. We explore what possible futures you might need to prepare for, disasters as well as triumphs. A life-planning exploration gives you the opportunity to imagine what your ideal future would be. Finally, we offer some suggestions about how to build long-term trust and confidence in your self and your relationship.

Final thoughts

Our own relationship has been a journey of discovery since it began five years ago. Our purpose in writing *How to stay in love* is to give you a guide to exploring the territory of your own relationship.

It is not easy. You may well find parts of each other's characters, fantasies and ways of looking at the world that seem threatening or unacceptable. But, in the long term, it will certainly be a fascinating and worthwhile exploration.

With your maps and compasses at the ready, you may now proceed.

Communication

Do you and your partner communicate? Of course you do. You talk about lots of things, all the time.

But do you *really* communicate? Communication is about more than just exchanging words; it is about sharing what is really going on inside you; it is about listening to what is really going on inside your partner.

We seem to believe that communication comes naturally. Certainly, when we are born we communicate skilfully and easily with the adults who care for us. We make our needs known by vocalizing in a very direct way; we drink in the sounds and movements of those around us and start to make sense of them. But then we get locked in our own shell; it is easier not to take in all the signals that other people put out to us, easier to ignore what people are trying to say. We try to communicate our true feelings to those around us, and are told that 'boys don't cry' or that 'it's unfeminine to get angry'. We see few adults around us really listening or really being heard. So we follow their example, and restrict our communication to surface matters, our job, the practicalities of life. Communication becomes a one-way affair—we transmit but no one receives. We feel misunderstood because we *are* misunderstood. The people around us feel misunderstood simply because we don't understand them, although we may think we do.

It's often true that at the start of a relationship, we find a new joy in communicating. We delight in every word our partner utters—and his tone of voice, and his every movement. But soon, the harsh world intrudes and we can easily get distracted by needs of day-to-day survival and find ourselves mysteriously failing to communicate again.

True communication?

Do you remember the last time you *really* felt heard or the last time you *really* listened? It may have been only this morning but it may have been a while ago. Remember that particular brand of attention you received and gave, the particular ease and safety with which you were able to make your real thoughts known. Wasn't it good? Wasn't everything else much easier because of that communication?

We believe that true communication between partners happens when you are safe enough with each other to really say what is really on your mind, threatening or not, when you are both secure enough in yourselves to really notice what is going on, what your partner's body is saying, as well as his words; what he is not saying, but wants to. Perhaps true communication is listening long enough to work out how to get what you both want out of a situation rather than just meeting the needs of the person who says most.

Communication is a loop

One of the main things we have learned is that communication is a *looped* activity. It is a bit like getting the giggles—one of you starts and both of you end up rolling round the floor. If one of you takes a step forward and communicates clearly and effectively, you both begin to communicate better.

Alternatively, if one of you stops communicating, or gets angry and lashes out, then the other will often follow suit. The system can spiral downwards or upwards equally quickly. This is why many of the explorations in this chapter are about increasing your own ways of communicating as individuals—about getting the skills to notice more, to be clearer, to take risks. If you do so, you will find that you communicate better.

The explorations

The explorations in this chapter deal with a variety of ways of communicating more skilfully in a number of situations.

- **Reading the signs** What subtle non-verbal cues do you and your partner exchange? They probably tell you more than words, and understanding them can give you deep insights into each other. This exploration gives you practice in noticing and interpreting them.
- **What do you *really* mean?** As we explained in the introduction, we often use the same words but have different meanings for them. This may cause distress because effectively you are in different worlds without realizing it. We help you learn to understand each other's real meanings for key concepts.
- **Getting what you both want** Most communication between partners involves explaining what each wants—and many major disagreements result when these wants conflict. This exploration gives you the basics of negotiation. With these, you can work towards meeting both your needs—a key element to the survival and development of any relationship.
- **What might happen?** Some thoughts and feelings are very personal and you feel scared to share them. You have been conditioned to believe that it is weak to be scared, threatening to be angry. The first step is to consider what you are afraid might happen if you *do* share your true feelings. Then you can go on to make sure you can cope if the worst comes to the worst.
- **Breaking the news** Once you are ready to share risky communications, you need the framework to do so. This exploration helps you identify the best times, places and ways to talk about difficult issues. In doing this you can also begin to explore your feelings around the issues themselves.
- **What I really want to say is . . .** Sometimes, it just seems impossible to say what you want to your partner. These pages give you writing space in which to put down your real thoughts and feelings before deciding how to tackle your partner face to face.

What next?

If you work through all these explorations, or the ones relevant to you, you will then have begun to explore some of the most basic issues in your relationship. Whatever is wrong, communicating will help change it. If the communication ceases, or becomes dishonest, then your partnership is indeed in trouble.

On the other hand, the more able you are to communicate what is going well, the more able you are to continue the happiness which is your right.

Exploration 3 — Reading the signs

You probably know the signs that tell you your partner feels one way or another already. Is he happy, sad or angry? Does he know when you're bored? You can tell by the way each of you moves, talks—or don't talk—what sort of a mood either of you are in. A shrug of the shoulders, a movement of the eyes or a particular tone of voice—all these are signals you should look out for.

You may know the signals already but you may not have thought about what they really mean. Body cues are not simply there by coincidence. Every subtle cue is really the outward sign, not only of an emotion, but also of an inward *need*—to be cuddled, left alone, talked to, or even rowed with!

The exploration

We've provided you with a simple drawing of a figure. Around it are various needs that you might have as you interact. You can add more if you think of them. (If your partner wants to do this exploration too, you can copy the page.)

Mark in on the drawing some of the ways your partner has of signalling his or her needs to you. You can use your own marking system to indicate just what you mean.

What sort of things should you mark in? What body cues do you notice? The main ones are often on the face—eye movements, mouth movements, perhaps even a change in colour as your partner feels irritated or uncomfortable, but a shift of the body, or a tapping toe can give you a signal too, as can a change in the rhythm or tone of voice. Indicate as many as you can, for as many needs as you can. To help, we've included our version of this exploration, with Sue showing Ian how she looks when she needs to be comforted.

Afterwards

What did you learn about each other? What new things—about the body cues, or about the real needs they signal—did you find out?

It's interesting to talk these through with each other, maybe finding out how your partner *really* feels when he looks that particular way.

The real impact of this exploration is not so much learning to notice the cues, as realizing what they really mean. If you can begin to recognize when your partner is signalling that he has need of you—or he can begin to recognize when you are signalling your need of him, then your relationship will immediately begin to reflect this increased awareness.

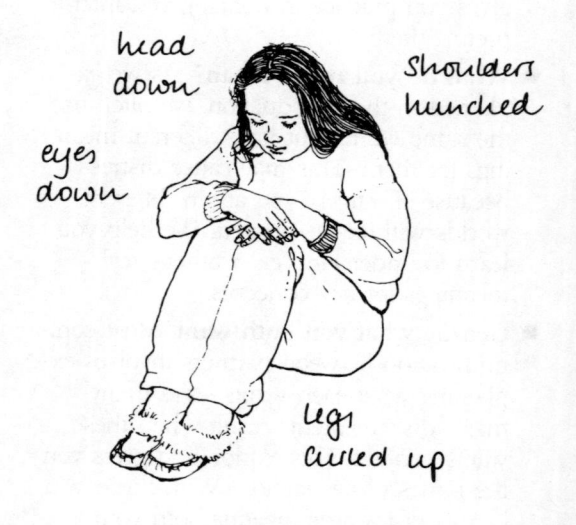

Sue needing to be comforted

Talked to

Listened to

Talked out of
something

Talked into
something

Taken seriously

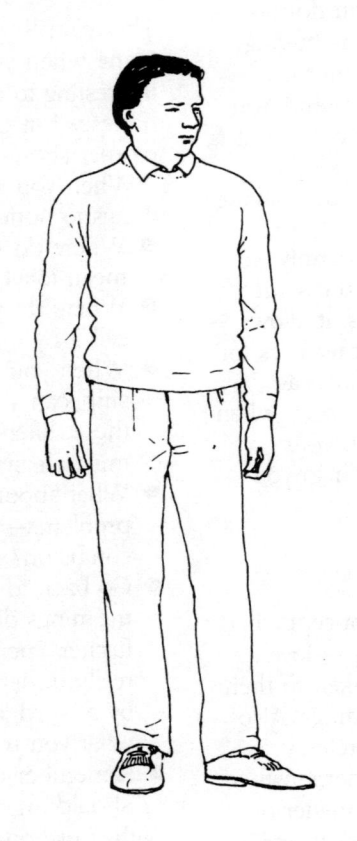

Cuddled

Played with

Left alone

Exploration 4

What do you *really* mean?

For any couple, concepts such as 'love', 'honesty' and 'trust' are likely to be important.

But when you use these words, do you both mean the same thing? Some of the worst problems can be caused when you don't— when for you, 'commitment' means buying a house together, while for your partner it means buying you a Christmas present! You may both use the word 'commitment', but it is really only a label, put on to such totally different concepts that you are actually talking about vastly differing world views.

This exploration allows you to identify ahead of time when you will use the same word—but do very different things. It allows you to learn what labels your partner uses for things that are important to you, such as 'love', 'freedom', 'honesty', so you know when you really have an agreement from your partner about the things that matter to you.

The exploration

The drawing shows some basic concepts that are important in many relationships—love, honesty, commitment, respect. Linked to them are some ways of showing these things. Also linked to them are some empty circles.

For each, fill in what *you* do to demonstrate this concept. Is honesty for you a matter of always telling the truth —or of never telling a lie? There's a great deal of difference. And what is your way of showing love? Commitment? Respect? Then get your partner to do the same, filling in what he does.

You can use the empty circles at the bottom of the diagram to choose other concepts that are important to you, and write in how you show those too.

Afterwards

The main learning from this exploration will come when you compare notes. It is interesting to note down how you show honesty, but comparing that with how your partner shows it is twice as fascinating.

When you are doing this, here are some things to notice and to ask yourselves.
- Where do you use the same words, but mean totally different things?
- Where do you mean the same thing, but call it by a different label?
- When you think back over your relationship, can you remember any times when these differences have caused misunderstandings?
- What about times when they have caused problems—disillusionment, resentment, confusion?
- Go back to the words where your meanings differ most, and discuss them further. Spend time until you feel that you really understand what your partner means by a word, and how it is different from what you mean.
- Remember that there is no blame. No one 'should' mean one particular thing when they use one particular word. The chances are that your partner does feel what you feel, but just calls it by a different name.

Finally, it's a good idea to revisit this exploration in a week or so. You may find that you have changed your mind about one or two things or realized something new.

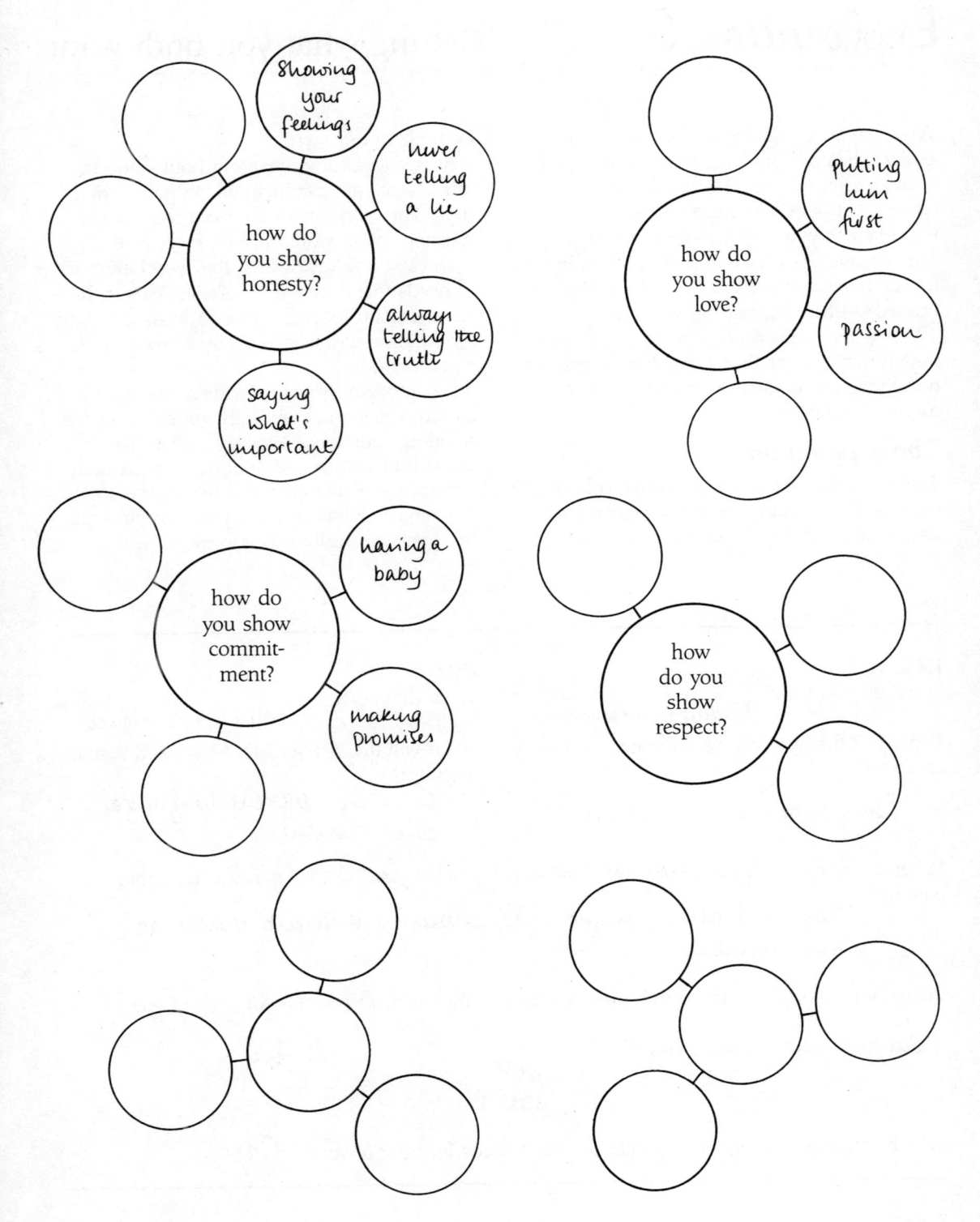

- how do you show honesty?
  - showing your feelings
  - never telling a lie
  - always telling the truth
  - saying what's important

- how do you show love?
  - putting him first
  - passion

- how do you show commitment?
  - having a baby
  - making promises

- how do you show respect?

Exploration 5 — Getting what you both want

What happens when you want something totally different from each other—a restaurant meal or a house move? What do you do when what is important to you is not important to your partner—and vice versa? This situation is very much the bottom line for many relationships. 'I wanted x and she wanted y—there seemed no way out.'

When this situation occurs, is there a way out? Perhaps it's neither a question of fighting nor giving in, but simply of communicating more effectively.

The exploration

There is a way, if you are prepared to keep talking, of negotiating a solution. Here's the format, followed by the exploration and an example of our own.

First state clearly what you both want. In our case it was seemingly incompatible holidays. Then, find out what need the want is meeting. What would having it get you?

Once you've established this, you have a list of needs that covers both of you. This is the starting point for negotiation. You have to find a solution that meets as many of your needs as you can.

If you begin by brainstorming, no holds barred, you'll come up with some impossible solutions, but some inspirations too. That could lead you to a solution that meets both your needs. Remember that the trick is to differentiate between what you want and the need you are really trying to meet.

HER
What do you want? *Holiday in Majorca*
What will that get you (i.e. what need is that meeting)?
Sun, relaxation, night life

HIM
What do you want? *Holiday in Florence*
What will that get you (i.e. what need is that meeting)?
Culture, different language and country

What are all the things you both want? What will that get you (all your needs, even if they conflict)?
Sun, relaxation, night life, culture, different language and country

Brainstorm possible solutions that meet as many of the needs as possible for both of you.

Sunbed and museums?   *Separate holidays?*   *Greece*

Which of these solutions would fulfil the most needs for both of you? *Greece*

HER
What do you want?

HIM
What do you want?

What will that get you (i.e. what need is that meeting)?

What will that get you (i.e. what need is that meeting)?

What are all the things you both want? What will that get you (all your needs, even if they conflict)?

Brainstorm possible solutions that meet as many of the needs as possible for both of you.

Which of these solutions would fulfil the most needs for both of you?

If you adopted that solution, what would happen? What would it be like? What would be the best thing that could happen?

Afterwards

This exploration gives you a format for working on your own issues. Taking our example as a model, use it next time you reach an impasse. Take your time to avoid getting irritated. If you both genuinely work towards meeting needs, you will both get what you want. The trick with this exploration is to do it every time you reach an impasse. In time, you won't need to do it deliberately—you will have picked up the strategy and will use it naturally and spontaneously whenever the situation arises.

Exploration 6

What might happen?

Often, communicating feelings can be easy. Sometimes, however, letting your partner know that you're angry or sad—or that you're happy when he's in a mood—can be very difficult.

What makes sharing such emotions difficult is fear of what might happen, for example, how your partner might react, what he might feel or how you would react to that. Often these are not real fears, but fear fantasy. If your partner would really be shattered if you ventured supportive criticism of his new shirt, then you are in deep water indeed. It is more likely that you are caught in a loop of stopping yourself expressing things because you have never had the courage to do so. Our fear fantasies come from a past when, as children, we were powerless, and were dependent on bigger, stronger adults. However, as adults ourselves, we have the resources to cope with what life throws at us.

The exploration

This exploration helps you think through what it is you are afraid of. This is one to do on your own, although you could talk it through with your partner afterwards.

The grid on the opposite page asks you to identify the emotion you are afraid of, and then to identify your three worst fears about what would happen if you did express that emotion. Then invent three possible ways you could handle it if each of your fear fantasies came true.

Afterwards

Doing this exploration may put you in touch with some valid fears. If you were to smash all the furniture, your partner might well leave you. On the other hand, it will also help you realize that many of your fears of expressing emotion are based on past messages, fantasies of not being able to handle the response.

It should also lay some ghosts to rest, as you begin to realize that you may now have the resources to face your fears and respond to them head on. Also, if you choose to discuss the exploration with your partner, you may well find that when checked out, many of your fears were totally unfounded.

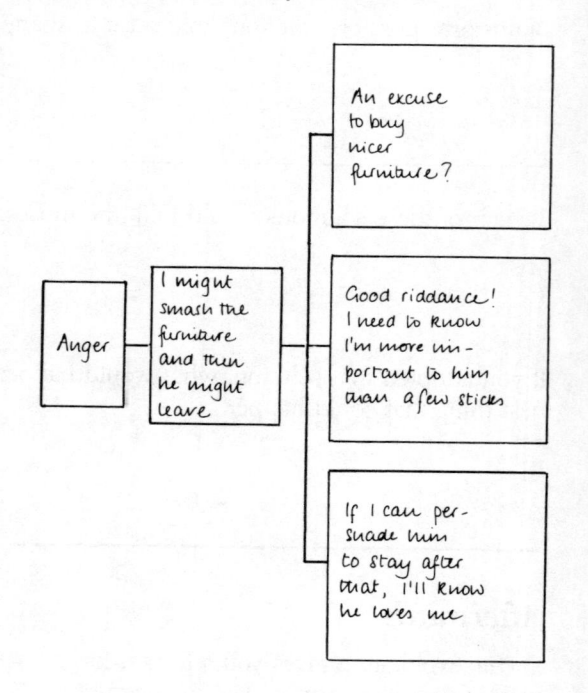

Anger	I might smash the furniture and then he might leave	An excuse to buy nicer furniture?
		Good riddance! I need to know I'm more important to him than a few sticks
		If I can persuade him to stay after that, I'll know he loves me

What is the emotion you don't want to express?

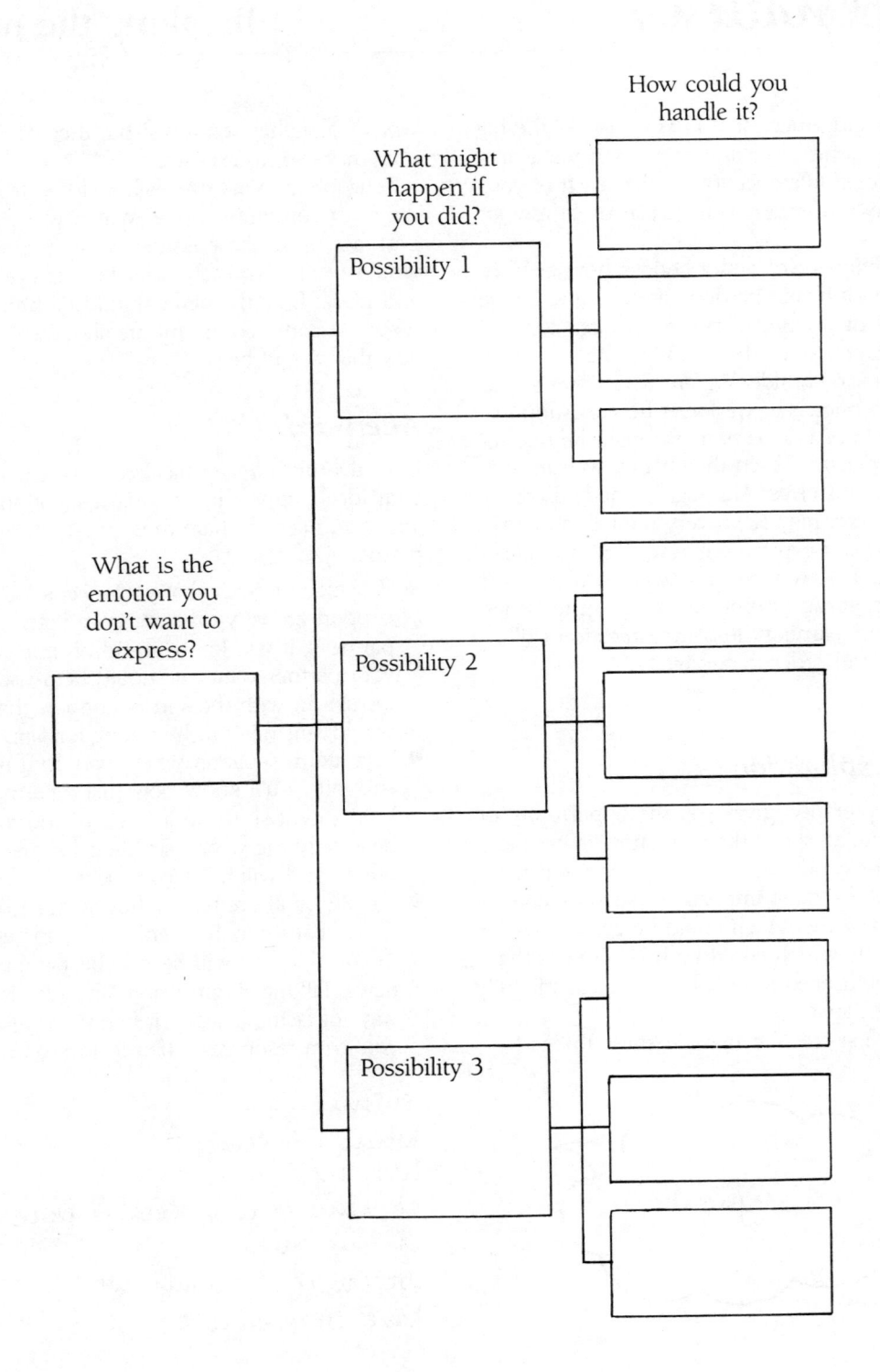

What might happen if you did?
- Possibility 1
- Possibility 2
- Possibility 3

How could you handle it?

Exploration 7

Breaking the news

When and where should you discuss the big issues? Time, place and mood can make an enormous difference to whether each of you is ready to discuss, to negotiate, or simply to listen.

Sometimes we cannot choose how news is broken—it has to be done at once and in the middle of a crowded street. Yet often we sabotage ourselves by choosing the wrong moment to confide. We are sometimes so overwhelmed that we forget how to support ourselves or our partners through the trauma or the delight. Given the chance, we *can* prepare ourselves. Although some bad (or good) news may seem very unlikely to happen, we can explore our reactions to it ahead of time. That way we can strengthen our partnership, ahead of time, by facing up to issues now, and learning the communication skills we need in order to survive.

The exploration

This exploration gives you the opportunity to work out, ahead of time, just how to set the scene for good communication. We've listed some of the most important issues we could think of, some which could be good news for you, some which could be bad, all ones that that would need to be talked through carefully and with love.

Your first reaction may be 'these things would never happen to us'. But they do, and they may—so no excuses.

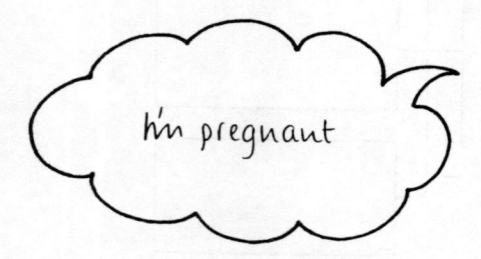

Your job is to talk through or to write down the exact conditions under which you could best face up to these issues: what support you would need from each other in terms of time and place; how the news should be broken; how you could communicate about it in a way that would help.

Afterwards

Even if your first step has been to write down your ideal support in important situations, you then need to share those with your partner.

- You may discover that your needs for support are very different from your partner's. If you know ahead of time what your partner wants, it should help you not to rush in with the sort of support that would suit *you*, but be wrong for *him*.
- In a future situation where you both need support, you'll know now that what may be the right situation for one of you may be exactly the wrong situation for the other—and will act accordingly.
- Finally, be aware that, although none of these crises may happen to you, sometime in your life you will have to bear important news. Talking about it now, and discussing ways of facing it when it happens will give you extra resources when it does occur.

(thought bubble:) I'm pregnant

(handwritten:)
Tell me...
when I'm relaxed;
happily;
at home or in a relaxed place;
on our own;
after work or when we have time to talk.

For me to tell you these things:

Where would be the best place?
When would be the best time?
When would be the best situation?
What state of mind would I be in?
How would you break the news?

- I'm pregnant
- I'm leaving you
- I've decided not to leave you
- I've had an affair
- One of the children is seriously ill
- One of the children has been arrested
- I've got the job
- I've been fired
- You're terminally ill
- I've crashed the car
- I'm terminally ill

Exploration 8 — What I really want to say is . . .

In every relationship there are times when things desperately need to be said but it's impossible to say them. Maybe that's because you are scared, maybe because it is no longer worth the trouble, you are not really saying what you need to say, and not really hearing what you need to hear.

At these times, you need some extra help.

Here is a space for you to write down what you really want to say, and also if it's relevant, write down what you are afraid you might hear. This is a space which makes it easier to communicate those difficult things.

The exploration

Don't leap into this exploration without some thought. Gather your resources. Remind yourself of any time in the past—in this relationship or an earlier one, recently or a long time ago—when saying what you really meant was worth it in the end. If you can think of more than one time, so much the better. Spend a few minutes reminding yourself of what you learned then—that being honest can have a positive result. If you want to write down what you remember, then there is space at the bottom of this page.

Then on your own, write in the spaces opposite what you think and feel. If both of you have things you need to say to each other, one of you will have to copy the page down. When you have finished, give what you have written to your partner, and both take time, apart from each other, to read and think about what the other person really wants to say. Remember that your partner is being as brave as you are in filling in this page.

Afterwards

Only when you have both had time to think about what you have both written, get together to talk.

This exercise is obviously useful in a crisis. If you really want to experience the power of it, however, do it when you feel a lull in your relationship, at one of those times when both good and bad feelings seem to be absent. The issues you bring up at times like this may well spark a row, but it clears the air like nothing else!

HIM	**HER**
When was the occasion when saying what you meant was worth it in the end? Where were you? What were you doing? Who else was there? What do you remember? And what did you lwarn?	When was the occasion when saying what you meant was worth it in the end? Where were you? What were you doing? Who else was there? What do you remember? And what did you learn?

What I think you want to say to me is . . .

What I really want you to say is . . .

What I think you want me to say is . . .

What I really want to say to you is . . .

Environment

When one is in a relationship that is an important part of one's life, it can be interesting to look at the effect your environment has on it.

What do we mean by *environment*? For the purposes of this chapter, we are thinking of it mainly as your home, because that is the part of your environment that you have most control over. We also include explorations on how you organize and maintain your environment.

Environment is important for many reasons. Firstly, environmental pressures can create strain. Many couples have serious problems trying to begin married life by living in mother-in-law's house rather than their own. Love may be able to flourish anywhere, but successful partnerships grow best when environmental pressures balance out.

Next, an environment in which you are both comfortable can allow you both to be yourselves and therefore happy in the relationship. Where the environment you set up does not allow you each to fulfill your needs, then strain will result. Not having enough space, enough time, enough comfort or enough colour can create destructive moods, and these will affect your relationship.

Creating your own special environment, your own home, can bring you closer together. Producing somewhere that expresses your relationship can teach you about yourselves and about each other. Having to create a harmonious balance between all your needs can teach you your first lessons in real negotiation.

Knowing what you want

The main block we have found couples meet in setting up and keeping their optimum environment is that of knowing what they really want. Outside elements, we are led to believe, are far less important than internal feelings. So if we feel in need of more space, more light, some heavy rock music or an evening in alone, we consider these as incidental. In fact, they can be very relevant to preserving a stable, happy relationship.

How do you find out what your real environmental needs are? The explorations we include in this chapter will help, but there are some ground rules, some of which are particular to this issue.

- Remember always to think about the environment you want in positive terms. It is far better to say, 'I want a really colourful room' than, 'No yellow . . .'. It's fairly difficult to decorate a room in 'no yellow'.
- It rarely works for one of you to design a place for two of you to live in. Both of you need to be happy, at least with the general idea, before you start. This is why many of the explorations in this chapter concentrate on working together to build ideas.
- Check out that the environment you choose is worth it to you. The mortgage may seem horrendous but it may be worthwhile; conversely, spending a year doing up a delapidated cottage may not be a valid way for you to be spending your time. You need to balance out all the costs—on your emotional bank balance,

as well as your actual bank balance—before committing yourself to a particular environment.

The explorations

The explorations we include cover a whole range of issues designed to help you design your most supportive environment.

- **Ideal environment** We begin by asking you to imagine your ideal environment— country, area, home. This helps you to think through your ideas freely before you begin to limit them. Identifying these ideals also helps you to think about what your real environmental needs are.
- **Creating a home** From the ideal to reality —using what you learned from the previous exploration, this one invites you to plan a home together. Negotiating to meet all your needs in detail, you can discuss the organization, furniture and decoration for an imaginary dwelling.
- **Creating emotional security** Your home environment will only work for you if it meets and supports your emotional needs. Which emotional needs do you expect to be met at home, and how can you organize your environment—sights, sounds, textures —to make you feel the way you want to?
- **Personal space** Many relationships founder because the partners consider they are not allowed enough 'personal space'. The problem arises when our different definitions of this very vague concept clash. By defining your own needs for personal space and comparing them with your partner's, you can begin to make sure that you are allowing each other the 'space' you both need.
- **Time together, time apart** How much time you need to spend together is a sub-division of the personal space issue. When expectations clash, real conflict can result; not least because, if one partner wants to spend less time with the other, it can be seen as a lack of love. This exploration helps you discover how much time each of you wants to spend with the other, and what this really means.
- **Division of labour** Maintaining your home is a joint responsibility, but is this responsibility equally shared? This exploration gives you a check list to work out who does what and whether you are both satisfied with this arrangement. If not, what can you do about it?
- **Tidiness** One partner's idea of 'tidy' can be the other partner's idea of cluttered. By working out your values and priorities about tidiness, and, in particular, whose responsibility it is to keep your place tidy, you can pre-empt many of the difficulties couples meet.

What next?

Once you have discovered what you need in order for your environment to be supportive, you may decide that you wish to put some of these ideas into practice. Whereas many of the other chapters suggest emotional developments or changes as the next step, this chapter could well lead on to practical steps in changing your home.

These steps do not have to be as dramatic as moving house—although we know one couple who did just that in order to give themselves a better environment in which to run their relationship. Simply changing the level of lighting, altering the washing-up rota or arranging to spend regular time talking when the children are in bed can create more comfortable interaction.

If there are deep and significant divisions in your relationship, then a new sofa will not cure them—but improving the quality of your home will almost certainly improve the quality of your relationship, too.

Exploration 9 — Ideal environment

Your environment can be your house, office, garden, neighbourhood, town—or even country. All these affect the way you feel—and thus the way you relate.

Here, we concentrate on the ideal. Why? Well, firstly because it would be nice if you didn't have to settle for less. Secondly because, with an ideal to aim for, you'll get further. So, for this exploration, go for an ideal. If you are working together, encourage each other to be truly outrageous in your demands.

Also, as with all the explorations in this book, it's worth noticing where the ideals differ—and working to give you both as much as possible of what you dream about.

The exploration

The facing page gives a number of questions for you to answer. It includes some space in which to write, though extra blank paper will probably come in useful if you really start getting enthusiastic about your plans.

You can work through the questions separately or together. If you choose to work together, you must accept your partner's right to express their fantasy. It does not have to be yours, and your ideal does not have to be your partner's.

Each question asks you to focus on a different aspect of your ideal environment: first the area, then more specific things until you have planned out a home in detail.

The exploration also includes questions designed to make you think about what is important to you. Is it the way your environment looks? Feels? Sounds? Is it important what other people think of it, does it matter what activities you do there? Whatever environment you choose for yourself in real life, it should fulfil these needs if it is to be really supportive for you.

You'll get most out of the exploration if you give your imagination a free rein. Choose your favourite shades, materials, shapes. Where you can, draw pictures, maps, plans.

If you are stuck for inspiration, remind each other of past memories that nearly approach the ideal 'You remember that holiday we had in . . .', or 'The attic room in that film was amazing . . .'. Talk through your ideal fantasy, *knowing* it is a fantasy and that you can enjoy it.

Afterwards

Having done this, you will certainly be more aware of what you want from an environment. In particular, focus on these things.

- How do your ideals differ—in space, place or activity?
- What needs do your ideals reflect—do you need privacy, security, a place to relax, or an environment that is buzzing with life?
- How are your needs different from those of your partner?

This may give you a great deal of food for thought. In order to create an environment that suits you both, you are going to have to meet many of those needs, even if they seem to conflict at first glance.

Remember, you don't have to have the same dreams in order to have a good future together.

Where in the world do you want to be—continent, country, area, town, district?

Imagine you are sending someone a picture postcard of where you live . . . what does it look like?

What kind of dwelling do you live in? Where would you work? What other places would you want to go to? For each, think about these questions.

- How will it look from the outside?

- What about the inside? Draw a plan.

For each room, described how it will look—size, shape, furniture, flooring, furnishing, colouring. How it will sound—what noises there will be as you move around? How it will feel as you walk or touch surfaces? How it will smell? Now describe the same thing about outside areas.

Who will you show your environment off to?

Who will be there to share it with you?

What will you do there—in each room, in the area surrounding your dwelling, in the neighbourhood, in the surrounding areas?

Exploration 10

Creating a home

Dreaming about your ideal environment may be fun. Using what you learn about your preferences to create a real home may be a little more difficult.

This exploration gives you the opportunity to use your preferences to plan an environment for your own use. It is not so much about home furnishing as about learning to work together to create the right surroundings for you and your relationship to flourish.

Her ideal—what she needs

His ideal—what he needs

The exploration

This exploration takes time and energy. You both need to have done Exploration 9, and from it, worked out what is really important to each of you. Jot down what you've found out in the space provided.

Next, look at the 'circular home' we've drawn out on the opposite page. (We've chosen it deliberately to be, probably, unlike the home you live in at present.) Imagine you've won this home in a competition. There's no cash alternative—you just have to live in it!

Work together planning the way you would organize, decorate and furnish this house. You can take it in turns to mark in your ideas (using a pencil so that you can change your minds) so long as the finished product is one you are both happy with.

Use the lists from Exploration 9 as a reminder of what it was you both said you needed in a home. Keep checking out that all your needs are being met, even if that means stopping to discuss (or argue!). If you end up with 15 sleeping spaces and no living room, that's fine if it is what you need.

Notice as you plan just how you work together to make decisions or to persuade each other to accept a particular idea.

Afterwards

When you have finished, ask yourselves these questions:

- What have you learnt about what you each want from a home? Do your needs clash? What could you do about this?
- What do you now feel you ought to think of first when planning or changing your home? What will you think of first next time you move house? Make two lists, in order of priority, one labelled 'essential' and the other labelled 'desirable'.
- If you were actually going to live in the circular home, and have it the way you have planned, who would be responsible for doing which jobs? What does that tell you about the way you allocate responsibility for building and maintaining your environment?

Kitchen

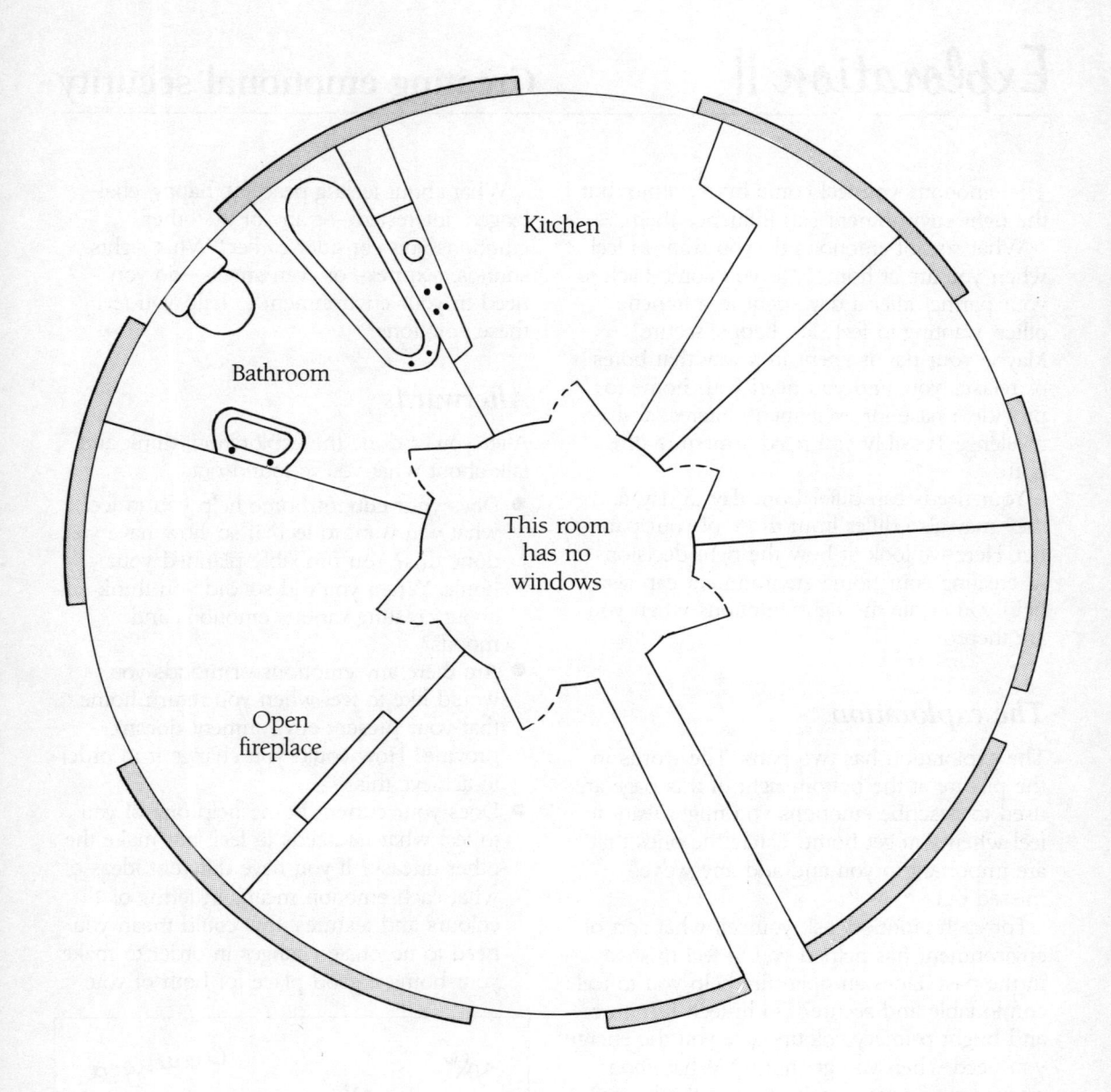

Bathroom

This room has no windows

Open fireplace

35

Exploration 11 — Creating emotional security

The emotions you feel come from within, but the right environment can influence them.

What sort of emotions do you want to feel when you are at home? Do you come back to your partner after a day spent in a frenetic office, wanting to feel safe, happy, secure? Maybe your day is spent in a way that bores or relaxes you, and you need your home to provide a base for excitement, interest and challenge. Possibly you need a mixture of both.

Your needs can differ from day to day, and they may also differ from those of your partner. Here we look at how the right decisions in creating your home environment can also help you create the right emotions when you are there.

The exploration

The exploration has two parts. The words in the picture at the bottom right of this page are used to describe emotions you might want to feel when you get home. Circle the ones that are important to you and add any we've missed out.

For each emotion, ask yourself what sort of environment has helped you to feel this way in the past. Does an open fire help you to feel comfortable and secure? Do hi-tech furniture and bright primary colours give you the energy you need when you get home? What about music, or favourite smells around the house?

The picture on the facing page shows the environment that one person chose in order to help him feel safe at home.

Experiment with drawing things *you* would need in order to feel safe—textures, sounds, visual elements. Your choice may be very different—you may need sharp colours, and bright lighting rather than dark corners and a cat.

What about feeling peaceful, happy, challenged, interested—or any of the other emotions you consider earlier? What sights, sounds, textures—or even smells—do you need in your environment to help you feel these emotions?

Afterwards

After you've done the exploration, think and talk about what you've found out.

- Does your current home help you to feel what you want to feel? If so, how have you done this? You probably planned your home. When you did so, did you think about creating various emotions and moods?
- Are there any emotions or moods you would like to feel when you return home that your present environment doesn't provide? How could you change it in order to achieve this?
- Does your current home help one of you to feel what he needs to feel, but make the other uneasy? If you have different ideas of what each emotion means in terms of colours and textures, this could mean you need to negotiate changes in order to make your home a good place for both of you.

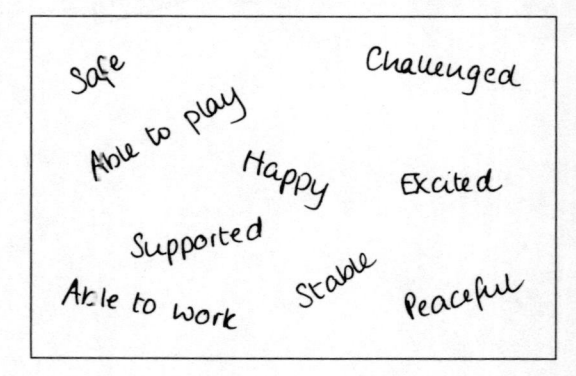

Safe   Challenged
Able to play
Happy   Excited
Supported
Able to work   Stable   Peaceful

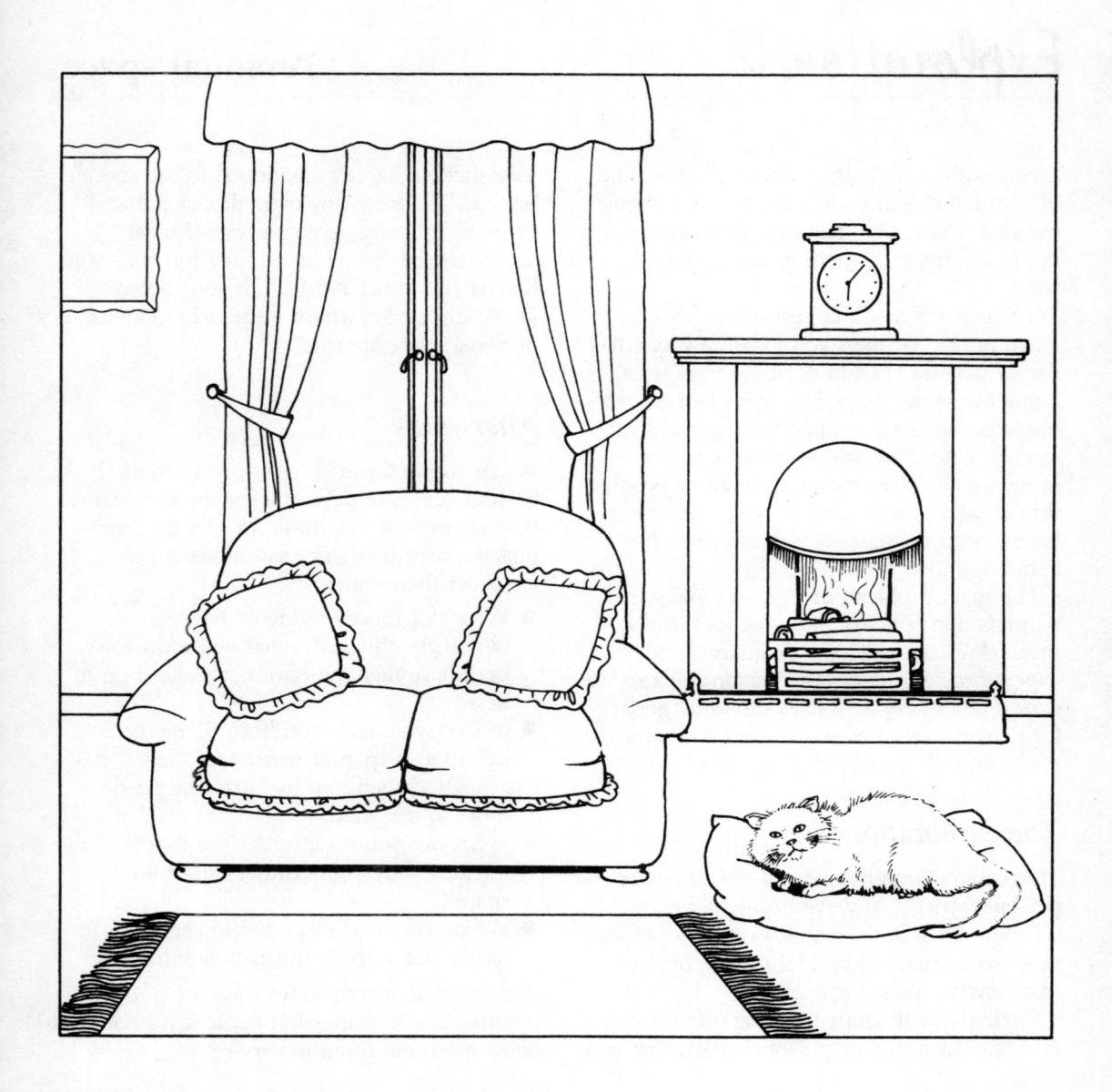

Exploration 12 — Personal space

Living with other people can be difficult, and often the problem is described as 'not enough personal space'. You may love someone dearly, but feel trapped by them in very practical ways.

It may seem as if the problem is your environment, perhaps you live in a very small flat, or need to spend lots of evenings together doing the same things, but very often, society has expectations of us just because we are 'in love'. Of course we will want to be in the same room all the time, meet the same people, do the same things. The fact that we often have a need for separateness can seem like a betrayal of love.

The main problem, though, is usually that partners don't understand what each other needs. We have our own definitions and expectations of the phrase 'personal space'. We expect other people to have the same needs for personal space as we do, and when they don't, we feel oppressed or rejected.

The exploration

This exploration gives several definitions of personal space that we've heard, all very different. Look at the phrases on the opposite page; some may mean a lot to you, others may have no meaning at all.

Circle the definitions that ring true for you. Add any meanings of 'personal space' that you have that we haven't mentioned in the speech bubbles. Jot down any extra thoughts that come to you, any developments of what you've circled. Think about why the ones you haven't circled are not real for you; do you know anyone for whom these definitions of personal space are true?

Afterwards

When you've finished, take time to think. If both of you have done this exploration, compare answers. If not, think about what you imagine your partner's answers would be. Consider these things:

- What differences suddenly become blindingly obvious? What needs do you both have that you have not realized up to now?
- In fact, what have you been doing (or not doing) to help your partner feel 'loved' has actually denied him the space he needs in order to feel good.
- What can you do in order not to feel threatened by your partner's need for space?
- What can you do in order to get your needs met without threatening him?

Remember that sometimes rows are not because love is dying—but because it's not being given the room to survive.

Twin beds

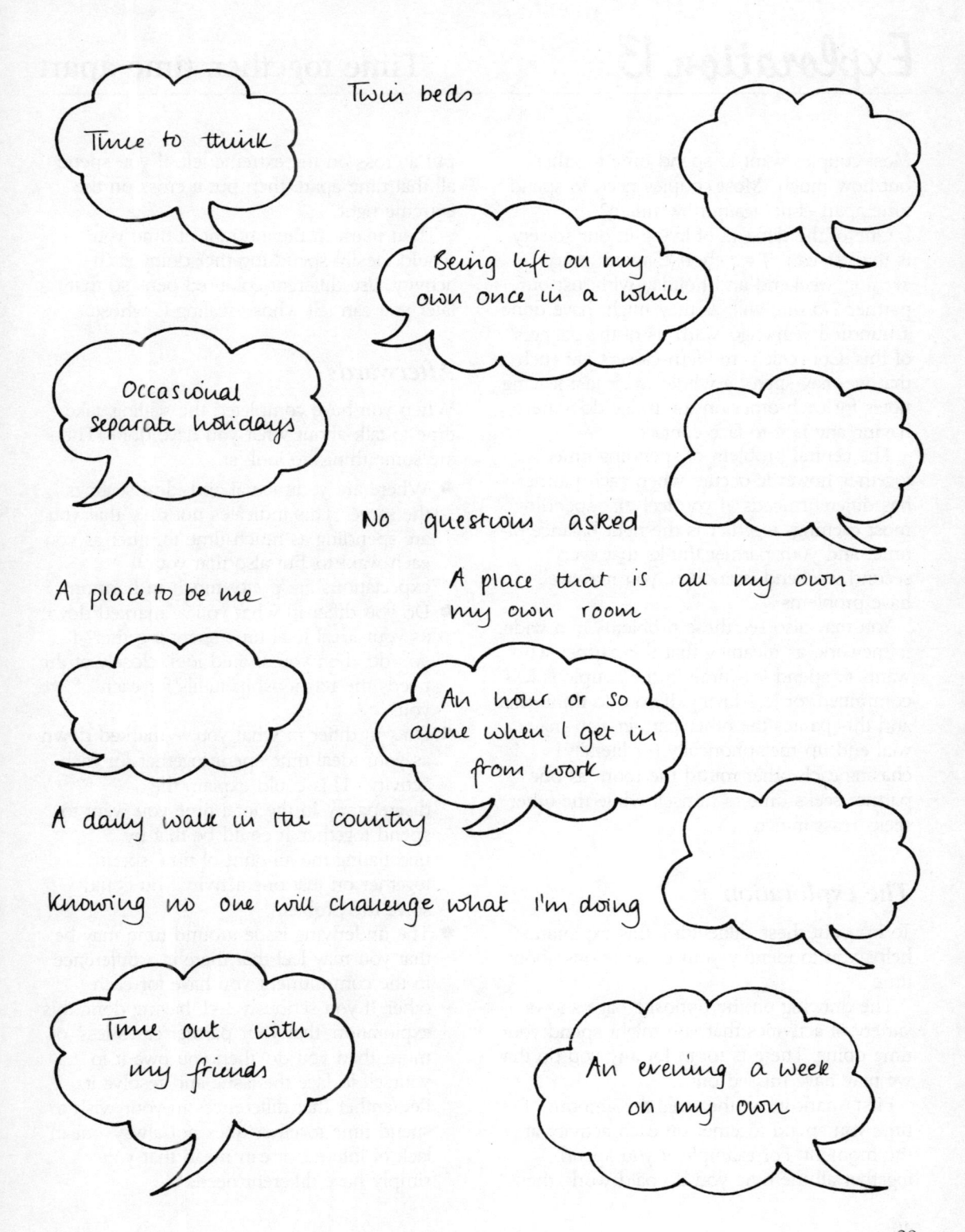

Time to think

Being left on my own once in a while

Occasional separate holidays

No questions asked

A place to be me

A place that is all my own — my own room

An hour or so alone when I get in from work

A daily walk in the country

Knowing no one will challenge what I'm doing

Time out with my friends

An evening a week on my own

Exploration 13

Time together, time apart

Most couples want to spend time together—but how much? Most couples need to spend time apart—but, again, how much?

One of the dangers of living in our society is that we can, if we choose, spend every evening, weekend and holiday with just our partner. No one will, as they might have done a hundred years ago, warn us of the dangers of this. Conversely, modern careers are such that we may spend a whole week just leaving notes for each other on the fridge door, never having any face-to-face contact.

The central problem of spending time together, however, occurs when each partner has different needs. If you feel that spending most evenings together is the right balance of time; and your partner thinks that every second weekend is enough, you may well have problems.

You may also see these problems in a wider framework, as meaning that the partner who wants to spend less time in the couple is less committed, or less loving. If you do think this, and this panics the other partner, you may well end up metaphorically (or literally) chasing each other round the room as one partner seeks time to himself while the other seeks reassurance.

The exploration

To iron out these difficulties, this exploration helps you to identify your expectations about time.

The drawing on the opposite page shows a variety of activities that you might spend your time doing. There is room for any you do that we may have missed out.

First, mark in on the scale the amount of time you spend together on each activity at the moment. For example, if you spend together all the time you do paid work, then put a cross on the extreme left. If you spend all that time apart, then put a cross on the extreme right.

Then mark in the amount of time you would ideally spend together doing each activity. Use different coloured pens so that later you can tell whose scaling is whose.

Afterwards

When you have completed the scaling, take time to talk about what you have done. These are some things to look at.

- Where are your actual and ideal scalings the same? This indicates not only that you are spending as much time together as you each want to, but also that your expectations are pretty much in harmony.
- Do you differ in what you've marked down as your ideal total time spent together? If you do, then you should look closely at the needs the relationship fulfils for each of you.
- Do you differ in what you've marked down as your ideal time spent together for each activity? This could explain the discrepancy in the total time you want to spend together. It could be that by negotiating the amount of time spent together on just one activity, you could solve the problem.
- The underlying issue around time may be that you may feel that there is a difference in the commitment you have for each other. If you seriously feel, having done this exploration, that your partner cares less, or more, than you do, then you owe it to yourself to face the issue and resolve it. Remember that differences in your wish to spend time together does not always mean lack of interest; it can mean that you simply have different needs.

	Always together **Always apart**

- Example (paid work)
- Spend weekends together
- Visiting
- Playing with children
- Changing the baby
- Watching TV
- Reading
- Walking
- Sitting in front of the fire
- Shopping
- Washing up
- Sex
- Voluntary work
- Sport
- Hobbies
- Holidays
- Work around the house

- Total time spent together

Exploration 14 — Division of labour

Who maintains your home? Be it housework, weeding the garden, keeping the kitchen knives out of the baby's reach—how does the labour divide?

In the old days it was easy; the woman stayed at home, the man earned the money. Now, arrangements can vary enormously from couple to couple. It really doesn't matter which arrangement you have as long as you are both happy with it and it works for you.

This exploration gives you the opportunity to take a long, hard look at the arrangement you have, how it works out in practice, and whether you're happy with it.

The exploration

This exploration can be done by either or both of you, but it's best if, when you do it, you do it separately, and cover in some way the section filled in by your partner. This is a real 'cheat's challenge'!

Read the list of tasks on the opposite page. Add in at the bottom of the list any jobs not mentioned that need to be done in your house. Then go through the list and mark an 0 in the column of the person who does each job. If both of you take turns, then mark 0 in both columns or, particularly if it's an issue for you, mark in the percentage of time each person does the job.

Then go back and put a tick where you are happy with the arrangement as it is.

Afterwards

When you've completed the chart, look over it. If you have both done the exploration, you may want to take time separately to think about it, or you may want to look at both sets of answers together. It's important to remember that the object of this exploration is to point out where you see things differently, and if you are unhappy about that. So be prepared for major differences of opinion and gasps of astonishment and horror as you realize that your partner feels just as overworked as you do!

- First, look at where there are ticks—where you are happy with what is happening. These are the areas where your system is working.
- It is where there are no ticks that you have to look closely at what is happening. What exactly is your dissatisfaction? What would you rather was happening?
- If both of you have done the exploration, also look at where you see things differently. Do you feel you always do the washing up, while he feels he always does? You might like to talk about your different viewpoints. However, there is no problem unless there is no tick. So look particularly carefully at areas you disagree on and are not happy with.

What can you do if you are not happy, particularly if your partner simply cannot see things the way you do? Here are some suggestions:

- Look at past messages about division of labour. Were you or your partner brought up to believe different rules —that 'men do all the heavy work' as opposed to 'women do their share'? You may like to swap expectations.
- Is the issue of housework masking deeper issues about who puts more emotional energy into the partnership?
- You can also solve housework issues in very practical ways. One married couple we know got home-helps and child minders from year one. It meant they went without other things, but their marriage *did* survive as an equal partnership.

	Her thoughts Jobs done by			His thoughts Jobs done by		
	Me	Him	OK	Her	Me	OK
Cleaning General cleaning Kitchen Fridge Cooker Toilet Carpet shampooing Windows						
Tidying General Bedmaking						
Shopping Weekly Day-to-day						
Cooking						
Washing up						
Laundry Washing Ironing						
Children Looking after (day) Looking after (weekends) Disciplining Taking to school Going to school functions as parent						
Other living things Feeding pets Watering plants Gardening						
Home maintenance Sewing Decorating						
Car Petrol, oil Servicing Cleaning						
Total work done						

Exploration 15

Tidiness

With the possible exception of where you squeeze the toothpaste, tidiness (or lack of it) and housework are probably responsible for more screaming matches than any other single factor. You would think that the odd beer can in the bathroom could not stand in the way of true love. In fact, the 'trivial matter' of tidiness can be the most destructive of a relationship, simply because it occurs so frequently. The underlying cause is usually a difference of expectation in one of three areas—who tidies, when to tidy and, most importantly, what counts as tidy.

The exploration

The exploration comes in two parts. First, look at the illustrations of a rather bare room. In one, draw the kind of things it needs until, in your eyes, it feels cosy. Get your partner to do the same with the other illustration. Now compare your pictures and use them as a basis to mark your opinions on the scale.

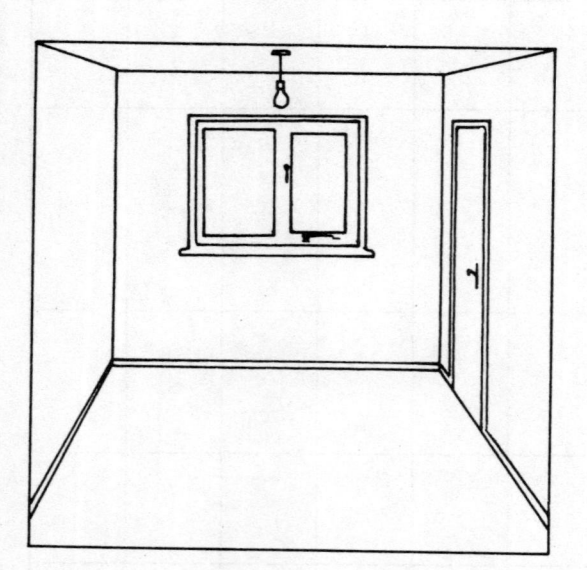

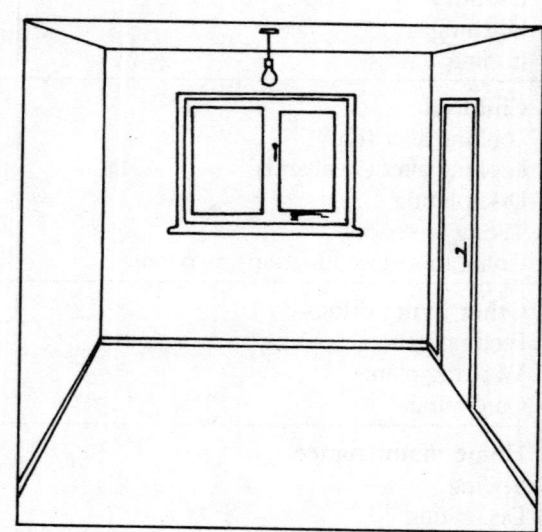

What is too spartan and what is too cluttered for each of you?

Totally bare room ──────────────── Not an inch of spare space

Where does something have to be before it is tidied?

Locked away out of sight ──────────────── Anywhere to hand

When does a room really need to be tidied?

When one thing is out of place ──────────────── When you can't move for clutter

Most of us are still brought up to expect that men create clutter and women tidy it. Who should do how much tidying?

Woman does it all ──────────────── Man does it all

Afterwards

Remember that your answers are what you would *like* to believe. The underlying attitudes of both of you may really be quite different, so you should only use this exploration as a starting point for discussion.

You will need to talk more about how you would like your home to be, and what makes tidiness—or clutter—important to you. When you find differences between you, you will want to start looking for ways around them. Here are some solutions we have come across:

- Nag him until death (or divorce) do you part.
- Have blazing rows about it.
- Do it all yourself and resent it.
- Designate separate spaces you are each responsible for.
- Divide the tasks between you.
- Get someone else to do it.
- Turn tidying into an enjoyable activity you can do together.

Other people

An intimate relationship can seem to be a world of its own, where you are isolated from the rest of the human race, safe in your own magic bubble.

In fact, from the very first time you meet, other people are affecting your partnership. You come to your partner the product of a whole lifetime of relationships with family, friends and colleagues. As time passes, you may well then choose to integrate your family and social life with that of your partner. The web of people within which you move affects your intimacy and is affected by it.

Past relationships

As we have pointed out throughout this book, past events affect the present. Whatever your past experiences have been, they will form your present expectations and the way you react. In no context is this more true than in the area of dealing with other people, beginning with your earliest relationships with your parents, proceeding through battles with siblings and school friendships. First loves, and later lovers—all of these will give you ideas about other people, men, women, couples and love. All of these will affect the way you relate.

Remember, however, that you are not the only person to be affected like this. Everyone else you meet has the same influences—but with each of them the end result is different. So while you are happy to take on your partner and all his past, you are also taking on a whole host of other pasts, biases and prejudices along with his family and his friends—as he is with yours.

Pushes and pulls

This may lead to problems. You may be totally at ease with the thought that your partner is the way he is. Your family, however, with their particular ways of looking at the world, may object to his sense of humour—or his job, or the fact that he didn't go to college. His friends, meanwhile, may consider you a drain on his energy, the girl who stops him from going down to the club with them on a Saturday night.

Just because you are now a partnership and want to commit yourselves to each other does not mean that other people will cease to have claims on you. In order to create a working relationship, you will have to make room for their demands, as well as maintaining your partnership as you want it to be.

Often, the simplest answer is just to remove yourself from the situation. Many people lose their social life because the pull of an intimate relationship is stronger than the demands of friends. Sometimes it's not so easy. You probably don't want to cut all ties with your parents so you need to work out ways of making sure your own needs are being met, that the partnership is growing, and that other people are being cared for as well.

This is where a supportive relationship can

help. Being aware that your partner does want to continue to show his love for his father, or to keep up the friendship with his best friends from school can enhance rather than threaten the commitment you have for each other by allowing each of you to follow your heart.

But sometimes you have to put your foot down. The bottom line, particularly where families are concerned, is that you are your own person, committed to your own relationship. You may feel a responsibility to other people, but if you bow to too many pressures, and allow too many people to make demands, you will lose sight of what you want for yourself, or even who you are.

The explorations

The explorations we offer in this chapter are all about balancing the needs and demands of other people with the needs and demands of your relationship.

- **Family tree** Looking at your family and your partner's family may allow you to gain many insights into your partnership. This exploration gives you a format in which to do this. You will not only learn about their expectations, hopes and fears of you and your relationship, you will also begin to understand a little more of how you and your partner gained your attitudes to such issues as being a couple; living together; marriage; having children.
- **Who do we go to for Christmas?** The seemingly small issue of how to spend major holidays and the more generalized issue of how to divide time between families, can, in fact, be a problem in relationships for years. The exploration invites you to consider family demands and the ways they conflict, and then to look at the needs behind these demands. In what ways could you meet the needs of everyone involved in the situation, particularly yourself?
- **Long-term responsibilities** For most families, there is a sense of responsibility for its members when they are in trouble. How does this affect your partnership? Will you be willing to help to look after your partner's widowed mother? What would he do if the situation was reversed? By thinking about these issues now, you can begin to explore your own and your partner's attitudes and plan ahead for these long-term responsibilities.
- **Your friends or mine?** Friends can form a supportive group that gives meaning to your life; so what happens when you form another relationship—that with your partner—that fulfils the same function? Different people find different solutions, and problems only arise when what is actually happening is not what you really want to happen. This exploration looks at how, as a couple, you arrange your separate, or joint social lives; and whether this is the way you want it to be.

What next?

These explorations only look at the tip of the iceberg. There are numerous other crises that can occur when other people's demands clash with those of the partnership.

The key is to use the basic concepts which we have examined in this chapter and apply them to any situation.

- What are the demands or issues involved?
- What are the real needs which these demands are hiding?
- What resources do you need to work out a solution that meets most of the needs of most people, without compromising your own integrity?

This sequence can be hard, but it is the basis of arbitration. And when you take on a partnership, and become caught up in the web of relationships that are involved, arbitration may be the key skill you need!

Exploration 16

Family tree

When you join a partnership, you often join a family too. Even if it only involves swapping Christmas cards once a year, you will be affected.

Each individual in the family will have his or her own attitudes and opinions—about men, women, relationships, marriage, children —and about the sort of person you and your partner are. So don't be surprised if you sometimes feel in the middle of a whole range of thoughts, feelings and expectations coming from your family and your partner's.

Sometimes they can be helpful—many new marriages have benefitted from the support of a close family system. But, sometimes, families can put a great deal of pressure on your relationship.

The exploration

The picture shows two blank family trees, one for each of you. Your family structures may contain a lot more members or a lot fewer. Alter the family tree until it looks right, and mark in the names of the important family members. Then write in what each person might be thinking about relationships in general and yours in particular. Think not only of what they've actually said, but of things you've heard them say about their own partnership, other partnerships, the roles of men and women, husband and wife, couples in general. For each person, find a key sentence which sums up their attitude, and which you feel probably influences the way they behave towards you.

Once you've completed the family trees, you need to look for general patterns within each family. Ask this sort of question:

- How does each family treat women in general? Men? Couples?
- What do you know about your family and what has happened to the people in it? What past experiences could explain why they feel the way they do?
- What can you as individuals, and as a couple, expect from the family?
- What will the family expect from you, and how will they react if you don't?
- What benefits can you think of of being part of this family? What disadvantages can you think of?

Afterwards

What can you do to optimize your family situation? Make the best of the advantages; even an overpowering family can have its good points; for example, it might offer a superb support system if one of you is ill. Make the best of the disadvantages as well.

- Keep reminding yourselves that your families' attitudes are from the past and really nothing to do with you.
- Remind each family that you are now a couple; their values and expectations are not yours.
- Learn to support your partner when he has problems with your family. Teach your partner to support you when you have problems with his.
- Agree with your partner how much contact you want with each family. Make sure you are both happy with this, then put it into practice. If necessary, write to each family telling them what your new contract with them will be and then be ruthless about enforcing these limits, right from the very beginning. You can always ease up if you get on better with your partner's family than you thought you would, but you cannot easily withdraw commitment once it is given.

HER FAMILY

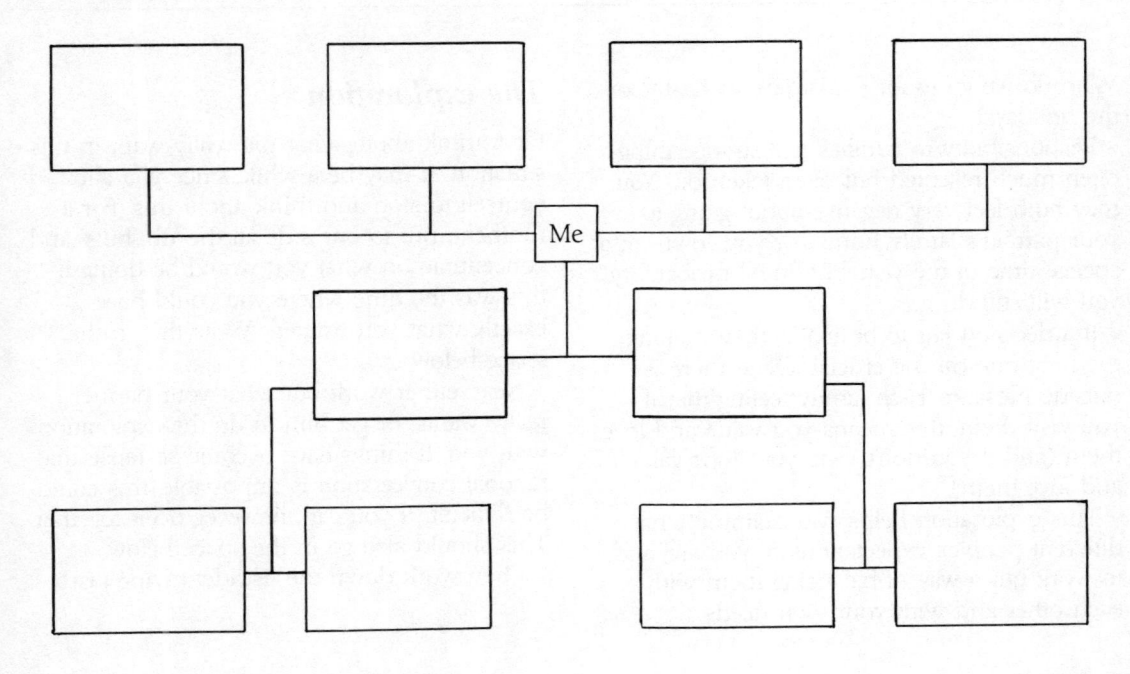

HIS FAMILY

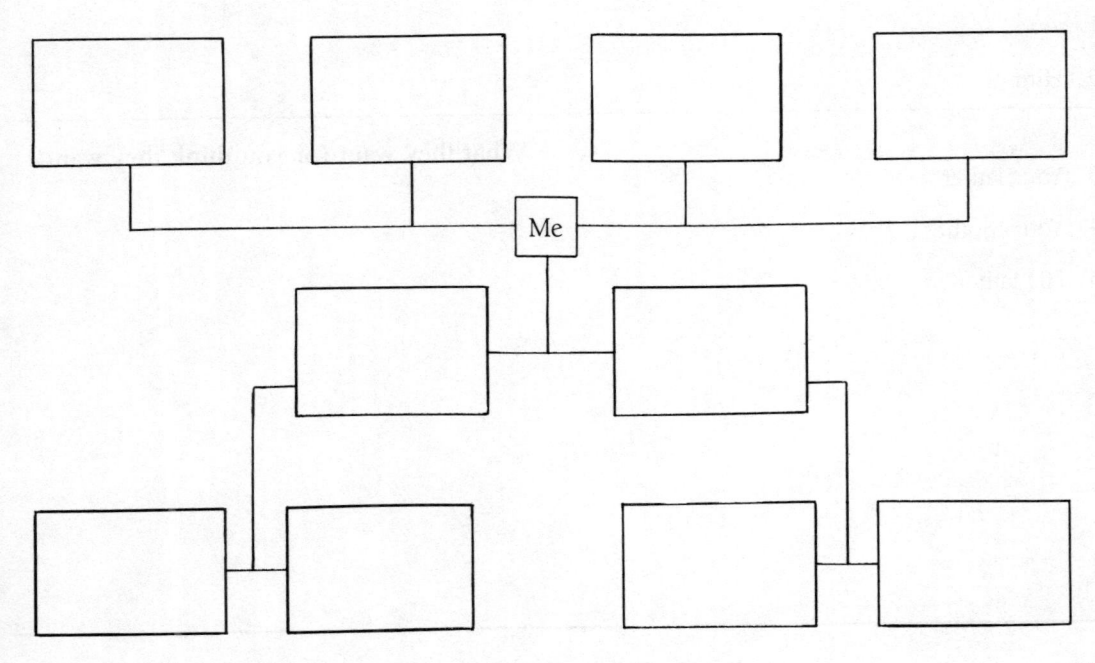

Exploration 17 — Who do we go to for Christmas?

Who do we go to for Christmas, or Easter, or the holidays?

Responsibility to families is a strange thing, often much resented but often taken on. You may both feel very negative about going to your partner's family home (or your own) at a special time of the year, but, in all probability, you will still do it.

If a decision *has* to be made, then making the right one can be crucial. Often there is outside pressure, each family feeling that if you visit them, this means you value and love them (and if you don't visit, you don't value and love them).

This exploration helps you examine what different people's expectations of you are, and to work out a way of balancing them with each other and with your own needs.

The exploration

First, think about what *you* really want in this situation. It may be a while since you allowed yourself to stop and think about this. For a moment, put to one side all the 'oh, buts' and concentrate on what you would be doing if this was the time where you could have exactly what you wanted. Write this in the space below.

Next, either work out what your partner really wants, or get him to do the exploration with you. If things have become so tense that rational conversation is impossible, this could be difficult. If you can, however, do it together. This should also go in the space below.

Then work down the list identifying just

People concerned

1 You

2 Him

What you want

What they want (or you think they want)

3 Your father

4 Your mother

5 His father

6

7

8

9

10

11

what each of the people involved wants. Fill in the relevant people's names—we've started you off.

Once you've filled in the grid, you will be left with a list of needs. Some may seem natural ('Of course Dad wants company on his birthday . . .'), others may seem outrageous ('They expect us to travel all that way just so that . . .') It may also seem that all these needs are totally incompatible. How can you go to both sets of parents when they live at opposite ends of the country?

Before you panic, think of the needs behind the demands. Your Dad may be saying that he needs you to be there to carve the turkey, but what he really needs is to feel that you are supporting him. Your Auntie Gertie may say that the kids will be disappointed if you're not there when what she really needs is to feel loved. Once you have realized that there is a desire to be acknowledged and loved behind all these needs, then you may begin to be able to see other ways of meeting these needs. What other ways could you help your Dad feel supported? What other ways could Auntie Gertie feel really cared for?

In the space below, brainstorm ways you could find of meeting the real needs of everyone on your list—including you. For the moment, include any idea, however silly. What about flying Concorde, and seeing everyone for two and a half minutes each?

Concorde to everyone . . .

Buy a videophone . . .

Afterwards

Once you've written down *all* your ideas look at your results. Most of them will be daft, but some may have the germ of an idea. Remember that what you are aiming for is some realistic way to show everyone that their deepest needs are important to you.

Use the brainstorm to develop three realistic, practical ideas. Remember that as well as meeting everyone else's needs, they must meet yours as well. After all, if you don't look after yourself, how do you expect anyone else to look after you?

Realistic Idea 1

Realistic Idea 2

Realistic Idea 3

Exploration 18 — Long-term responsibilities

What are your long-term responsibilities to your family, and to your partner's family?

Often, as you form your partnership, such things seem far off in the future, but if you have an awareness that, one day, they may be important, this will help you prepare for such an eventuality if it comes.

For example, what would you do if your partner wanted you to give his widowed father a home? How would he respond if your sister's children were orphaned and you were the only suitable people to look after them? Your response may be wariness—or welcome—but one thing is certain; your response will never be straightforward. You will always feel a variety of things when faced with such a big, long-term responsibility which, in some respects, you are not really prepared for.

The exploration

This exploration gives you an opportunity to think through some of the conflicting thoughts and feelings that may come up if you consider such long-term prospects.

Read the list of possibilities. For each, take the appropriate line on the grid opposite. In the first column, fill in your first reaction to that possibility. Be honest. If your reaction to the thought of your Mum coming to live with you is 'total horror', write that. Then think again. Is that all you feel? Perhaps there are emotions other than horror. There's pity, perhaps, for your mother. Concern for your partner. Write that down in the second column.

Keep going along the column allowing different reactions to strike you until you reach the least one. Take your time. Some of your true thoughts and feelings may take a while to surface. Go through the same process with all the other possibilities. Add on at the end any other eventualities that may be a possibility for you in your particular family situation.

Afterwards

When you've finished the exploration, you won't have any definitive answers, but you will have a great deal of information—about your conflicting thoughts and feelings, about which possibilities would be worst for you and which you could cope with.

If you partner has filled the grid in too, you will also know his varying thoughts and feelings. And they may conflict with yours.

What you do then is up to you. You may feel that most of these possibilities are so unlikely that they don't need talking about. Certainly, of the thousands of things that could occur in your life, these are only a few. The important, underlying thing is, whichever of them do crop up, you and your partner will need to understand each other's attitudes in order to be able to work with them. What is your partner's idea of responsibility? What limits does he place on it—towards your family, towards his family?

Understanding and accepting your individual concepts of responsibility can teach you a lot about each other, and make it easier for you to handle such responsibilities in the future.

Possibility	First thought	Second thought	Third thought	Fourth thought	Fifth thought
1					
2					
3					
4					
5					
6					
7					
8					
9					
10					

Possibilities to consider
1. Your father has died, and your mother wants to come to live with you.
2. Your partner's father has died and his mother wants to come to live with you.
3. Your mother has died and your father wants to come to live with you.
4. Your partner's mother has died and his father wants to come to live with you.
5. One of your/his family asks for the loan of a large sum of money that is the exact amount of your savings.
6. One of your/his family has died, leaving two children to be looked after.
7. One of your/his parents is terminally ill and needs home nursing.
8. One of your/his family is housebound and wants you to go and live with them.

Exploration 19

Your friends or mine?

Your partner may be your best friend, but the chances are that you will need other friends too, in order to live the life you want to. This raises a whole series of questions: When you have a relationship, do you carry on your social life just as before? Do you expect your partner to get on with your friends, or vice versa? Do you expect to get on with your partner's friends?

At the bottom of this page is a 'map' of a couple and their social life, as seen by one partner. She has drawn in the way she sees her partner and herself, and the way she sees them relating with their friends. Around the drawing, she's written in some explanations and other thoughts she had.

The exploration

Draw your own 'social life' map. It can take a different form from Gill's; you can choose any way you like of expressing what is happening in your social life. Take your time and write down any thoughts you have while doing it. Then think about how you would like your social life to be ideally. Which friends would you want to see? How often? Doing which activities? Draw another map to show this.

Afterwards

When you've done this, you may want to think about some of these things.

What is your social life like? Are you happy with the way it is? In particular, do you hanker after the sort of social life you used to have before you formed your partnership?

Negotiating a different social life can bring up spectres of all sorts—jealousy, insecurity and infidelity. It may be hard to say, or hear, that your partner wants to spend time with other people. Here are some things to think about while you are negotiating:

- The social life your partner had when you met helped to make them the person you fell in love with, so why knock it?
- The social life you had when you met your partner helped to make you the person you are, too.
- Wanting other friends doesn't mean you don't love your partner.
- Not getting on with your partner's friends doesn't mean you don't love your partner.
- Having other friends may make you more interesting to your partner, and vice versa.
- Spending time with friends does not mean having an affair (unless having an affair is what you really want . . .).

If both of you have done the exploration, you need to examine where you differ in the way you see things, and, of course, where you differ in how far away from your ideal the reality is.

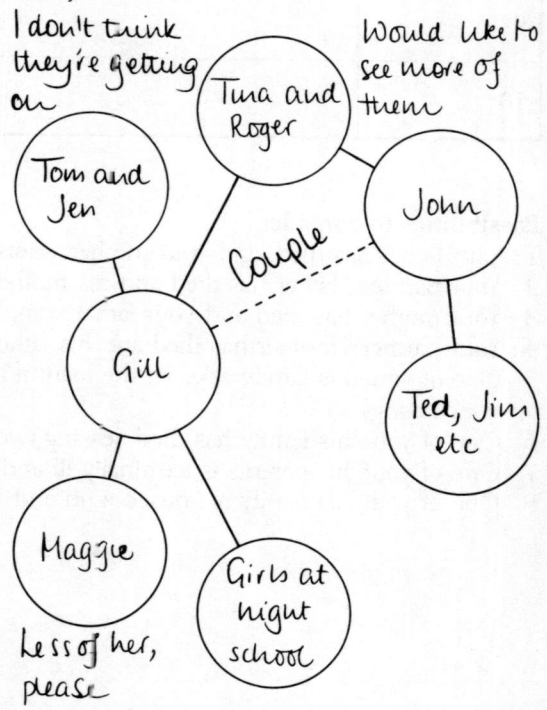

HER
Friends—the way it is

Friends—the way I'd like it to be

HIM
Friends—the way it is

Friends—the way I'd like it to be

Work

Times change, and in particular, views of work change. Over the last few decades, there has been a revolution in who works and how; in the way we see work; where we expect to be when we are working; in how we expect work to fit in with raising our families.

Whereas years ago the work roles fulfilled by each gender were clearly defined, they are now blurred. For example, it can well be the woman who earns the chief salary. Recently, it has become more acceptable for men to stay at home and take a more active role in child rearing or home maintenance. The whole shift towards flexible working hours, fewer working hours, as well as the increase in unemployment means that the old standard of 'nine-to-five' may well soon be a thing of the past. 'Leisure' is now a growing industry, and our leisure hours form an increasingly important part of our lives.

This may mean that you and your partner come to your relationship with very different ideas of what your working lives will be like. It is essential to explore these differences, in ideas and expectations, and be clear about the issues around work—and around play.

What's the ideal?

At best, work, play, family, outside interests and your relationships should fit neatly into your life appropriately and complement each other. Ideally, you would both be able to have the career you want; you would be able to start and stop working when you wished, sharing child care as appropriate; money would simply not be a problem.

Many of these ideals may not be possible because of outside factors. The present employment situation and the renewed pressure on women to stay at home can challenge any couple's ability to plan their lives the way they want. However, you can have control over *your* attitudes and feelings—particularly those about each other. There can be real acknowledgement of your partnership in the way you trust each other about money. You can be flexible and tolerant about the pressures on a partner who stays at home, or one who goes out to work.

The secret of success

It seems that one of the key elements of success where the issue of work is concerned is that of *values*. Because of changing views of work, we have changing values. One of you may see supreme value in career achievement while the other still regards work as a 40-hour-per-week way of paying for the skiing holiday. It is here that many crises arise.

Whenever something that someone does is not valued, either because it is not regarded as difficult, or because it's not being rewarded by money or by positive emotion, you are likely to get problems. Resentments can arise and defensiveness creep in simply because there is a mismatch between what someone does and how much someone else values it. Conversely, if you both work and play in ways that both of you consider valuable, you are likely to have a more satisfying relationship.

The explorations

All the explorations we include focus in some way on making sure you understand what each of you values. They all challenge whether you value and reward the activities of both of you throughout your relationship.

- **Work and play** Our definitions of work and play can differ enormously, as can the value we put on each. This can lead to major complications when you attempt to set up a relationship which contains within it both work and leisure activities. The first exploration looks at what judgements you and those around you make about these things. These can threaten your relationship by creating an inequality. How can this be resolved?
- **Working together** Whether or not you share the same career, you will work together at some point in your partnership—painting the hall or arranging a holiday. But, because you are different, and because you place value on different skills and abilities, working together may cause conflict. Irritation, jealousy, competitiveness can all undermine your effectiveness. This exploration helps you to identify your differences and see the value in them.
- **Financial equality** The most obvious result of work is money. The way you handle money can reflect the structure you have in your relationship and the value you put on each other's contributions. This exploration helps you identify what your money arrangements say about your relationship, and check whether this is really the way you want things to be.
- **Staying at home** Whether by choice or necessity, one or both of you will probably stay at home at some time during your relationship. This can cause stress both on the partner who stays at home and the one who does not. This exploration encourages you to find out how you feel when you are together, having spent such different days, and makes suggestions about how to cope with the problems which can arise from this.
- **Life plan** It is important to be aware of your expectations about career, family and the way you will spend your life. This exploration gives you each a chance to identify key stages in your life and that of your family and to allow you to talk about their respective value ahead of time. In this way, you can begin to plan so that potential clashes of interest can be planned for.

What next?

If you do lay the foundations for a really good working life within your relationship, by supporting each other to do what you really want and by placing value on activities for their own sake, you may find this has other benefits. You may find that not only does your relationship improve, but that your activities—paid work, leisure, home-building—also become more enjoyable. If, as a partnership, you can really integrate your working lives into your 'loving' lives, then you will change both.

Ultimately, too, the goal should be to mix work and play to such an extent that we are always choosing to do what we enjoy. It may seem an ideal—but it is worth aiming towards, and worth bearing in mind as we make our life choices.

Exploration 20

Work and play

What is work and what is play? Finding out which is which, at least in your relationship, can be crucial to its success.

Our society thinks of work as necessary, and play as unnecessary. We tend to put higher value on things that earn money and think that anything that involves spending money is therefore less worthwhile. These attitudes can put pressure on a couple which is trying to combine work, play, paid activity and unpaid activity in an attempt to live their lives harmoniously. If you think that any activity that isn't paid is worthless, and he enjoys helping out at the youth club twice a week, you might end up arguing.

Other people's opinions may disrupt you too. Does his mother think that having a family is more worthwhile than your high-flying management job in industry? Do your women friends think you're letting the side down by staying at home and looking after the children? Does your family criticize him for going out with his mates?

Find out what you each regard as work and what as play, and then let this lead on to a discussion about the intrinsic value of what you each do. You each in your own way contribute to the relationship, but it might be that you, or he, or other people that affect your relationship, see some activities as more worthwhile than others.

The exploration

The exploration lists a variety of activities. If we've missed some that are an important part of your life, put them in the empty spaces at the bottom of the grid.

The shaded line indicates a variety of opinions, from considering each activity to be completely 'work', to considering it to be all 'play'. Mark your view of each activity.

Ask your partner to do the same, using a different colour of pen, and if there are any people in your life (your boss, his Mum, mutual friends) who you think have opinions about this which may affect your relationship, then mark in their opinions too.

Afterwards

Which issues do you have differing views about? Which other people have views that differ from yours? In what ways could these differences cause problems?

- One of you sees the other's activities as 'play', not serious work. Try swapping roles one weekend, and find out how much 'work' you really do.

- One of you resents the other's 'playtime': hobbies or relaxation. Remember, even if you are *seriously* short of money, everyone needs time to relax in order to stay sane.

- One of you is unhappy in their work. Can you really afford to change? Can you really afford not to, if you are to give each other a happy life? Look at what you can do to retrain for a job which will make you happier, while the other partner gives support for a while. Failing that, what can you do to make the miserable one's leisure hours as fulfilling as possible?

- Other people's opinions maybe masking a division between you. Check whether you are actually in agreement about how you divide your time between work and play as a partnership. If you are, and are happy with this, then either ignore others (even if they are close family) or tell them to mind their own business.

To what extent is each activity...	Work ──────────── Play
Daydreaming	
Paid job you like	
Paid job you hate	
Voluntary job	
Housework	
Looking after children	
Evening job in a bar	
Playing sport	
Overtime	
Buying clothes for work	
Business lunches	
Work-related social activities	
Shopping for house	
DIY	

Finally, remember that a playful attitude to work means more creativity, more motivation, less stress for you as individuals *and* as a partnership. Look back at the list of activities.

What would your life be like if you could honestly mark every one of them at the play end of the scale?

Exploration 21

Working together

If you choose not only to be emotional partners, but also working partners, you are choosing a very difficult path. Even if you do not work together in your careers, the chances are that you spend time together working on joint projects—building a home, raising children, perhaps getting involved in some sport or hobby. These can be an integral part of building a relationship together, but there are a number of dangers involved with this.

Spending too much time together in one of these and you may like to look closely at Exploration 13 (on time together, time apart). When you work together, particularly if you live together as well, you need to be wary of driving each other up the wall—or boring each other rigid—just because you are in each other's company so much of the time.

Another problem can be confusion of roles. If you have an issue with a colleague, then you can usually be professional enough to regard it as just one of those things, but if the person you disagree with is also the person you love, then the arguments, disagreements and negotiation take on a personal edge, and both work and emotional life suffer.

The ways in which you are different can provide an important key to understanding a working partnership. These areas can form your greatest source of strength, because you complement each other professionally as well as personally. However, they can also create competition, rivalry and jealousy. It is a good idea to identify them—and begin to appreciate them—as soon as you can.

The exploration

Fill in the chart opposite. Think of any areas you can in which you are different from each other. It isn't only the obvious differences that matter, like physical strength or being able to speak a second language—what about the more subtle ones, such as making phone calls, writing letters or raising the energy in a meeting?

Afterwards

When you have filled in the chart, discuss it with each other.

- What are your differences, the places where your different skills are based on different ways of thinking, acting, and looking at the world?
- Notice the places where it is easy to accept and feel good about your differences. If you feel close and accepting, build on this!
- Notice, too, the areas where you may feel threatened by difference. Why doesn't your partner do things the way you do? You may feel put down by this—or jealous of it. You may simply feel very irritated. If you feel competitive, use that to spur you both on to greater efforts.
- Can you now, over the next week or so, start to become aware of how your differences, the places where you each have strengths, actually strengthen your partnership? How do they turn you into a winning team rather than a losing compromise?

.... is better than .... at

1 Physical strength
2 Organization
3 Communicating
4 Raising energy
5 Creativity
6
7
8

.... is better than .... at

1 Physical strength
2 Organization
3 Communicating
4 Raising energy
5 Creativity
6
7
8

Exploration 22 — Money

Ever since money was invented, control over the money supply has always been an issue for families, and before that, they argued over goats!

Do you have separate bank accounts? Joint bank accounts? Separate accounts but with a joint account for joint expenditure? There is no one 'normal arrangement', so you must make your own decisions as a couple. The real issue is not what solution you choose, but whether you are both happy with it.

The control of money can often be a reflection of the general pattern of control within a relationship. So if your arrangements about money truly reflect the balance of control you want in the relationship, then you will be happy with them. If they somehow contradict this balance of control, then there will be a basic conflict in your situation and problems may arise.

The exploration

The exploration contains a number of questions for you to answer. The first part asks you to identify the principles by which you arrange your finances. This can be difficult to do—and you may find that you are unclear, or disagree about the principles, even though you have a working financial arrangement.

The second section asks you to work out which practical financial arrangement most reflects your principles.

- If you believe in equal control, you will most likely have some form of joint account—or a mechanism by which equal money can be taken out of a joint fund.
- If spending and earning power are linked, you need to have some way of operating this, often by having separate accounts.
- If equal control plus a degree of autonomy is your goal, you may well have a joint account plus separate accounts.
- There are many other ways of organizing your finances, which may reflect the many other possible balances of control. Remember, too, that situations can change—couples who begin by having separate accounts can move into having joint accounts, and vice versa.

Remember, joint bank accounts are not necessarily a sign of a closer relationship.

Part 3 of the exploration invites you to consider whether you are happy with your actual financial arrangements, and whether it reflects your negotiated agreement.

Afterwards

If your actual arrangements do not agree with your principles you may want to change them. Remember that there is no point in negotiating a new *financial* deal unless you agree on the *emotional* deal behind it, so first make sure that you are both absolutely happy about what your principles are.

Then negotiate hard and carefully for a new financial arrangement that reflects this.

Part 1

What principle would you say most nearly describes your attitude to money within the relationship?

Discuss this until you have an agreement. Here are some suggestions:

- We have an equal relationship, so we have equal control of all the money.
- We have different responsibilities within the relationship, so we each control different amounts of money, from different sources.
- It's no different from before we met.
- From each according to their abilities; to each according to their need.
- We share, but place limits on spending that reflect how much we trust each other or ourselves with money.

Part 2

Once you have decided on the principle upon which your money issues are concerned, look at these ways of operating your finances. Which of them would most accurately reflect the principles you have identified in Part 1 as being behind your attitudes to money?

- Joint account
- Separate accounts
- Joint accounts with separate accounts
- One account in one person's name
- Joint account with credit card in one person's name
- Other

By what rules, if any, would you operate this system?

Part 3

Think again. Look back at Part 2. Which financial arrangement do you actually operate? Is it the same as the one you have identified as reflecting your principles?

Is your current financial arrangement one you are totally happy with? Do you need to modify it by putting in upper limits on spending, or changing to a different bank account arrangement? Would you really be happy working out your finances in this way? Check out the slightest niggle, or it will rebound on you later.

Exploration 23 — Staying at home

What happens when one of you is staying at home? It may be because you have chosen to do so, to look after your family, or to do some studying. It may be that jobs are hard to find and you have no choice. It may be that one partner places a lot of value on the other partner 'not having to work', and so insists on it.

Years ago, it was the norm for one partner to stay at home. Women had other women to chat to and to share experiences with. This is now the exception, and there is little or no support from the outside world—particularly for men who stay at home.

There can be such a difference between the way you each spend your time that you may begin to feel separated, or resentful. Society puts a great deal of emphasis on one's identity being tied up with one's job, so being a 'house wife' can make you feel inferior.

The exploration

Look at the words on the opposite page and think of how you feel in the evening, when you are together but have spent the day apart, doing different things.

Circle the words that you associate with the way you feel. Get your partner to do the same with a different coloured pen. If other words seem appropriate add those too.

Afterwards

When you've both done this, look at the results. Obviously if you are both happy and contented then count your blessings. But if not, there may be some stiff negotiating to be done. It is actually easier if both of you are unhappy with the situation, as then you will both be committed to changing it. If only one of you is restless, the other may be tempted to press for keeping things as they are. Remember that money issues ('I know you don't like the job, but what about the mortgage . . .') can seem all-important, but you—and your relationship—may well be happier in the long run with a slight drop in income and a more contented life.

The section on page 22 about negotiations could well help here, as you try to find a solution that works. To start you off, here are some solutions to these issues that we've heard of couples using. They might start you thinking . . .

- Role swap: partner A works, partner B child-minds.
- The stay-at-home partner goes to work, but uses the salary to 'replace' themselves with a child-minder and home help.
- One partner takes a lover.
- The stay-at-home forms a co-op with other stay-at-homes, to share work and give support.
- The stay-at-home works in a bar in the evenings while their partner child minds.
- The worker job-shares.
- The stay-at-home partner goes out a lot in the evening with friends.

```
                              Complete

    Frustrated


                    Empty
         Happy

                                    Tired
   Down



                  High energy


   Bored                          Fulfilled


                  Low energy


  Wound up                      Invigorated
```

Exploration 24 — Life plan

Your job, your family, things you want to do, ways in which you want to develop—all of these are a vital part of your life. And so is your relationship. Whether you are considering a long-term or a short-term partnership, thinking of how all the pieces fit together is a wise precaution.

Obviously you cannot know exactly how your life will develop. A pools win or a car crash can change everything overnight, but if you can identify how you would like to see things going in general terms, then you can plan for that and avoid possible conflicts.

The exploration

The lines on the opposite page represent your life and your partner's life. The central line represents the pattern of your family life. Children, or the possibility of parents coming to live with you should be marked on it.

The end of each line at the bottom of the page is the present. Mark in the current year there and number the stages up the line in five year gaps. Then each of you should mark in on your own line the following things:

- The year you will probably retire.
- Any key career changes, when they will probably happen or when you would like them to happen.
- Any times you would like to take courses, and at what time.
- Periods into or out of full-time work, because of children.
- Any other 'breaks' from normal work routine, such as travelling or study.

We are looking for thoughts such as, 'I'd like to do a degree, and I'd like to do it before I'm 40.' These thoughts will, of course, be very vague. Nevertheless, mark the sort of thing you would like to do, given the opportunity.

Then mark in on the central line some key stages in the lives of your children. How old are they now? When will they have all left home? When will they stop needing daytime and evening care? If you expect to have dependent relatives come to live with you at some time, mark that in too.

Afterwards

When you have finished, you will have a clear picture of your individual expectations of your family life over the coming years. This picture will show up areas of potential conflict, which will be much easier to deal with if you talk about them now, ahead of time.

- Is the career of one of you more important than the career of the other? What does that mean for the other one's life plan?
- Whose responsibility is child care or caring for older relatives? How will you arrange this? How will this be reflected in your career commitments?
- Will you expect to support each other through periods of study or time off?
- What will the bottom line be if one of you agrees to a joint life plan and then wants to change it?

Future (add in the dates)	Her life	Family life	His life
_____			
_____			
_____			
_____			
_____			
_____			
_____			
_____			
_____			
_____			
_____			
(Now)			

Feelings

Love, respect, admiration—and fear, hate, sorrow—we will probably experience a thousand feelings during the course of an intimate relationship. Many explorations in this book deal directly or indirectly with your feelings about separate topics—so why include a chapter specifically about them?

In this chapter we are looking at feelings that in one way or another are an issue on their own. Perhaps we don't have enough of them—such as self-esteem, or affection, or perhaps we believe we have too much of them—like irritation or boredom.

Where do they come from?

Where do feelings come from, and what controls them? The rush of adrenalin that accompanies anger or the relaxation that tells us we are feeling contented are physical symptoms. As new babies, we get them when Mummy doesn't feed us, or when she does. They are physical responses to physical stimuli, unhindered by 'shoulds' or 'shouldn'ts' about whether to feel them or not.

As we get older, two things happen. Firstly, we build up links which tell us when to feel emotions. The first time we burn our fingers, we do it because we didn't know to be cautious or afraid. The second time, we are cautious, and we don't get burned.

We also learn that some emotions are unacceptable and we are told 'It's wrong to get angry'; 'Boys don't cry'. Often we feel it, but don't express the feeling in words or actions.

Past events, present emotions

Learning these lessons as children helps us survive as adults, but it also presents us with problems. The links we make between trigger (like flame) and emotion (like fear) may be accurate they may also be inaccurate, particularly because, as adults, we have more control over our environment, and we have more skills than children.

So, if we learn at three to be afraid when Daddy shouts, we may still at thirty-three be unable to cope when someone raises their voice. If we learn at eight to be nice to Mummy if she's tired, we may confuse this emotion and end up placating our lovers. One major lesson to learn about your own actions, and those of your partner, is that, if you feel bad, it may not be what is happening *now* that is causing the problem. It may be that you are still influenced by past issues that have made you vulnerable. If your partner seems hurt, it may not be you but his past memories that are hurting him.

Remember that it is our past which creates us and makes us what we are. What irritates you may be totally acceptable to someone else—it is your particular set of experiences that makes you unique, and which also makes you vulnerable. Remembering this when you are in the middle of a screaming match can save your relationship. Being able to see the past as over and the future containing potentially totally different feelings can keep you sane.

The danger of not feeling

We learn as children that some feelings are not acceptable. We still feel them; the adrenalin still pumps, the excitement still rushes, but we don't show them because they upset the adults who control our lives. When we grow up, we still find difficulty in feeling those emotions. Sometimes, this causes stress-related problems, such as heart attacks or migraines—but it can wreck our health and our love lives.

In an intimate relationship, it is wonderful to feel the positive emotions of love, acceptance, joy, pride, as well as the 'negative' emotions such as grief, fear and anger that add depth to intimacy. If we've been trained not to feel these emotions, however, it's not easy to enjoy the fullness of our relationships. If you or your partner have learned through several years of childhood that people will be upset by too much emotion, you won't 'unlearn' that in the first week of a new relationship. If you can allow yourself to see emotion as unthreatening and encourage your partner to do the same, you will start to be able to feel.

The explorations

- **Self-esteem** The first exploration looks at our hesitation in being aware of our strengths. It encourages us to explore our identity in terms of what is good about us, and so begin to build our self-esteem.
- **Individual or partner?** Which is more important for you, feeling part of a couple or feeling that you are your own person? To maintain a balance, it can be important to look at your feelings about taking the other point of view.
- **Where are you vulnerable?** Past experiences can create trigger points which mean you react strongly to a voice-tone or a look on your partner's face. Identifying when this happens and what it means can help you have more control.
- **Creative rowing** A row may mean upset and disharmony, but it can also mean that you are both maintaining your identity within the relationship. Doing this exploration after a row can help you see the feelings in a different light and begin to use rows in a more constructive way.
- **Keeping boredom at bay** The saddest feeling in a relationship is boredom. This exploration investigates what you mean by boredom, and gives you the chance to identify what it would be like if your relationship became boring. What can you do to maintain the interest you once had?
- **Jealousy** If we feel that someone else is taking away the good things in a relationship that should rightfully be ours, we can get jealous. This exploration helps us to get things in perspective and take effective action.
- **Motivating each other** We can get upset and frustrated when our partner lacks the motivation to do something both you and he want. This exploration helps you to work out a positive way to motivate each other, using your own natural strategies.
- **In love forever** How do you keep the same sense of possibility that forms such a large part of being in love? This exploration provides a format within which you can communicate your hopes for the future and your support for those hopes.

What next

This chapter offers some basic ideas and practical actions so that you can begin to take charge of your feelings. It could be that, having started, you find whole new problems occurring. What happens to a man when he cries for the first time? How will you feel when you finally allow yourself to get angry? You may feel angry, frightened, or upset as you begin to find out about your emotions, but given the chance, your capacity for being joyous, happy, and euphoric will grow too.

Exploration 25 — Self-esteem

We are not the first people to point out that you have a better chance of building a good relationship if you have high self-esteem—in other words if you like yourself. It is worth putting quite a lot of time and energy into deliberately building your self-esteem. This exploration is just to start you off.

Before you start, you will need to consider what you think self-esteem actually is. It's all very well liking yourself, but just who or what *are* you? Very young children have no concept of self; it's something we develop only as we learn to apply labels to ourselves. The first is a name, 'I am Mary', then comes family membership, 'I am the daughter of the Smith family'. As we get older, we develop lots of others, identifying us by our social or ethnic group, 'I'm black'; by our occupation, 'I'm a computer programmer'; by our religion, 'I'm a Christian' and so on. We develop self-esteem by internalizing messages about how well or badly we fulfil each of these roles: 'I'm a *good* computer programmer'.

We often develop more sophisticated identities as well. We might, for example, identify ourselves most strongly by our past achievements, our imagined or expected futures or even our fantasies. We can build self-esteem by confirming that we are 'good' in any or all of these roles.

The exploration

In the first part of the exploration we have listed some statements of identity. Take a little time to step into each identity and find out how real it feels to you, then rank it from one to ten, ten being the one that feels as if it has least to do with who or what you are. If you like, you can add in others at this stage that also feel like important elements of your identify.

In the second part, write out your top three again in the left hand section of the grid. You could make them more specific at this stage. So, for example, you could put, 'I am a computer programmer' in place of 'I am what I do'. Then think of ways in which you are good in this identity. If you are doing the exploration together, this is the part where you can help each other most. Challenge each other to be specific, and give real examples of *exactly* what it is that makes you so good. Write these in the right-hand side of the grid. The act of remembering or imagining these positive aspects of your personality will build your self-esteem, so take your time! Incidentally, we are not suggesting that you should ignore aspects of yourself that you do not like—but they are not a part of this exploration.

Afterwards

There are lots of ways you can carry on this process after the exploration.

- If you keep a diary, make sure to write in what you have liked about yourself each day.
- Every morning, look in the mirror and tell yourself why you are good.
- Ask other people what they like, respect or think is good about you—but remember that these opinions only become self-esteem when you come to believe them yourself.
- You might have found this exploration difficult or disturbing. We often believe that social acceptance comes from putting ourselves down rather than celebrating ourselves. At this point, you must make your own decision about which outlook you want on life, and which will be better for your relationship. If you decide to

change, remember that a book is not a powerful enough tool to deal with strong distress. Use the resources section in the back as a starting point for finding a good counsellor or therapist.

Rank these statements in order, starting with the one that you least identify with.

I am my parent's daughter

I am what I have done

I am what I do

I am what I will do in the future

I am my job

I am my body

I am what I dream

I am what I believe

I am what other people think I am

I am the wife of my husband

Re-write your top three, being specific about your circumstances	How do you know that you're good at this?
1	
2	
3	

Exploration 26 — Individual or partner?

Do you think of yourself as an individual first, and a partner second? Or is it the other way round?

Your ideas about yourself can centre around what you do as an *individual*, the achievements you yourself create, your own personal friends and lifestyle. It can be that the most important thing for you is your identity as part of your couple, the home you make together, the relationship you are building. For most people, identity is made up of a complex mixture of the two parts of themselves—individual and partner.

The exploration

This exploration invites you to find out about that part of you you're not usually aware of. First you need to decide whether, usually, you identify most with yourself as an individual or as a partner. If it is difficult to decide, choose one at random. Then, concentrate on the other option—as an individual if you normally see yourself as part of a couple, as a partner if you are normally more aware of yourself as an individual.

Think particularly of yourself in this role. How do you feel? How do you think other people see you? How does your lover see you? What are the advantages of being in this role—the good things about it? Then think of the disadvantages. What do you miss out on? What can't you do?

Fill in the appropriate column of the grid with the advantages and disadvantages of the role that you normally don't take. Get your partner to do the same.

Afterwards

When both of you have filled in the grid, look at what you have written.

First, consider your realizations. Look at the advantages you've identified in the role opposite to the one you normally take. Maybe you usually cut yourself off from these. How could you incorporate some of them into your relationship? Then look at the differences in your roles. Does one of you form your identity mainly from being part of a couple and the other not? Perhaps this is causing some friction for you, when one wants to go everywhere together and the other wants to go out on his or her own. How could your realizations of the advantages of the other point of view help you understand each other—and go some way towards changing yourself? If you want some practice in the identity you don't usually take, then try some of these things.

If you normally see yourself as a partner:

- Try saying 'I' instead of we in conversation.
- Take off your wedding ring (or equivalent) for a day or two.
- Take a weekend away without your partner.
- Try doing something on your own that gives you a sense of achievement (hang-gliding, teaching a course, etc.).

If you normally see yourself as an individual:

- Try saying 'we' instead of 'I' in conversation.
- Wear a sign of your partnership, such as a ring, for a day or two.
- Include your partner in some of your individual activities.
- Spend time with your partner doing something that needs you to work co-operatively (rowing, riding a tandem, playing on a seesaw, singing harmonies together).

	Couple		Individual	
	Him	Her	Him	Her
Pros				
Cons				

Exploration 27

Where are you vulnerable?

You know the feeling. You may be quite happy, you may be a little emotional. Then, your partner says or does something that really gets to you. An immediate rush of anger —or euphoria, or boredom, or any strong feeling—hits you. 'Button pushing' happens when something your partner does or says triggers a strong emotional reaction in you, without any logical reason. Your partner wasn't trying to upset—or enthuse—you, but for some reason, you reacted strongly.

Why does this happen? What your partner has said or done, the way he has looked or the glance he has given you, has reminded some part of you, often unconscious, of a time in the past when you felt a strong emotion, so you feel that same emotion again. The past experience may be a result of your present relationship—a subconscious reminder of a time you had a terrible row. It may have nothing to do with what is happening now; early childhood memories of being shouted at will be even stronger than adult ones. Equally, a particularly gentle tone of voice may push very early pleasure buttons and remind you of very early cuddles!

There's no point in trying not to feel strongly—the very point of buttons is that you have no control over them when they are pushed. There's no point in your partner trying not to look or sound that way—that will only make things worse. What you can do is to become aware of your buttons, negative and positive.

The exploration

First, fill in the grid on the opposite page. Identify six buttons that your partner pushes for you: three negative and three positive. Fill in the grid with details of what your partner does to push those buttons, what behaviour, expression, voice tone. Add what the feeling is and where you feel it in your body (a rush of anger in your tummy, tension in your back). What does it mean? (I love you; you're getting at me; things are going wrong between us).

Afterwards

When you've identified the buttons, think about these things.

- For the negative ones, be particularly aware of the very first 'twinge' of emotion that tells you a button has been pushed. How could you, at that point, simply step outside the bad feeling?
- How could your partner realize that your buttons have just been pushed, and do something positive to 'unpush' them? What do you need your partner to say or do (tell you he loves you, give you a hug, steer clear of you for a few minutes) that would give you a chance to cope with this totally illogical emotion?
- When could you use the positive buttons in your relationship to make good times even better? If a particular endearment means a lot to you, and never fails to make you feel good, when could your partner use it to make a positive experience a euphoric one?

This is a very individual thing, and one which every couple needs to work out for themselves. Couples who are really aware of their negative buttons can soften their effects so fast that really powerful bad feelings never have time to build up. Couples who are adept with their positive buttons will press them repeatedly, building good feelings and bonding themselves closer together at every opportunity.

	What you do				What it means to me	How I feel	Where I feel it
	Action	Look on face	Tone of voice	How you touch			
Pleasure buttons							
Pain buttons							

Exploration 28 — Creative rowing

Rows can seem like the end of the world. Yet there are couples who row furiously—right to the end of happy, lifelong relationships. Other couples never say a cross word to each other, yet still have short-lived, unfulfilled partnerships.

It depends how you see it. Rows need not be seen as destructive and debilitating, but as constructive and creative. They can be a way of building respect, creating understanding and making a partnership more solid, if only we can learn from them. Rows arise because of differences between us, differences in what we want, what we feel, and in the way we see the world. These differences are rarely wrong in themselves—it is the mere *fact* of the difference that creates the row. These differences exist in virtually every relationship, whether or not that relationship features rows. In fact, it is these differences between us that create the original spark of interest and excitement that can later lead to love. When the differences lead to rows, we are simply experiencing the other side of the same coin.

This exploration is to help you discover that your rows can be a valid expression of your suitability for each other. They can also be a way of establishing your strength; developing a real partnership without domination or oppression.

The exploration

You can do this on your own, or together.

Just after you have your next row, try answering the questions on the opposite page, taking your time and thinking through your responses. You can either do it together, or spend time separately. Compare notes and discuss what you have discovered. Be aware of differences between you, and also of the strengths that the row has highlighted.

Afterwards

In the days that follow the row, continue to notice what your differences and strengths are. Remind each other of what you have learned that is useful and of the insights you have gained that you would never have had if it had not been for the row.

When you row again after that, notice how your view have changed and how you are beginning to use rowing as a way to build up, not knock down, your relationship.

What was the row about?

How would you have felt if you had got your way?

You could have avoided the row by giving in. How would you have felt about it if you had?

How would your partner have had to look at the issue in order to understand you?

How would you have had to look at the issue in order to understand your partner?

What deeply-held differences in values did the row express?

How are you stronger as a team because you are different in these ways?

Has this row enhanced your respect for each other? If it hasn't, go back and start it again until it does!

Exploration 29 — Keeping boredom at bay

One of the main reasons given for couples splitting up is boredom.

After years of living with, and learning about each other, the spark in a partnership can die. Day follows day with little difference and little excitement. Of course one partner or both can become restless—the famous 'seven-year itch', for example. Sometimes they decide that life is worth more than this, and, whether by forcing a break through a manufactured crisis, or simply letting a break happen through inertia, the partnership dissolves.

What causes boredom in relationships? Is it simply that, having spent ten years (or ten weeks) with the same person, we are ready for something new? Or is it that once we are in a partnership we stop developing and become boring ourselves?

The exploration

The first part of this exploration then is to ask yourselves what you mean by boredom and, having identified the feeling, think about what boredom would mean in your relationship, and what the signs are (falling asleep a lot, having an affair, getting irritable) that would tell you you were bored.

Once you have done this, compare your feelings; check that one person's idea of boredom isn't the other's idea of stability. If one of you is heading happily towards a quiet life while the other is trying to avoid it like the plague, you can expect problems. You need to understand each other's needs, and, by understanding, and perhaps negotiating, avoid letting one person's heaven turn into the other partner's hell.

Boredom may not just be about not staying in to watch television each evening. It may be that since you first met, neither of you has changed, and so you are both faced with a situation so stable that it is truly boring. There is nothing frightening about changing. If you watch children, you will find that they do it all the time, as they learn, grow, develop. Like children, we can change, learn new skills, take on new perspectives, and avoid the stagnant stability that kills relationships.

The second part of the exploration gives you a chance to list, first of all, three things your partner could do to during the next week to renew the excitement you created together at the beginning. Choose easy ones, such as going out for a meal, rather than deep ones such as, 'Please undergo a total personality change.' Then, list three things that you could do to change yourself. You don't have to wait for someone else to do it for you, you could learn a new skill, play a new role, be less punctual, or more unpredictable. Just for a week, just to keep the interest up.

Afterwards

The point is not what happens during that week, not whether you learn Japanese or take up skate-boarding. The point is not whether you both like what happens, or whether you row about it, it is to begin to realize that your relationship doesn't *have* to lapse into boredom. Things can change. And so can you.

Part 1
What sort of things (other than in the relationship) bore you? How do you feel when bored? What things do you do that tell you you're bored?

How would you know your relationship was getting boring? How would you feel? What would you be doing that would tell you you were bored? What things would you be scared might stay the same?

How would you know your partner was boring? How would you feel about him? In what ways would you react towards him that told you you were bored with him? What sort of things about him would make you scared in case they never changed?

How would you know you were becoming boring? What sort of things would you be doing, feeling, thinking? How might your partner react?

Part 2
List three things your partner could do during the next week to make life more interesting for you both.

List three things you could do over the next week to make life more interesting for you both.

Exploration 30 — Jealousy

The 'green-eyed monster' has been the subject of a multitude of books, films, romantic songs. But what is jealousy, and how can we recover from the emotion? If you feel that someone or something is taking away something that you expect to be yours—in this case, the good things you have in your relationship with your partner—then that is jealousy.

Jealousy isn't only about sex. You can be jealous of your mother-in-law if she monopolizes your husband's affection. You can be jealous of a sport, or a job, if you feel that it is taking away your partner's energy or attention.

The exploration

Use this exploration particularly if you are aware of feeling jealous of someone or something in your partner's life. Do the exploration alone, giving yourself the time and space to be really honest.

First, identify what it is you are jealous of. Then think about what it is that you feel is being taken away from you that you expect to be yours. Is it time, energy, love-making, or just Friday nights that you feel are your right? Write these down in the spaces provided opposite. Next, think through what your rights really are. This demands some honesty. Do you actually have a right to your partner's presence *every* evening? Is it your right to expect love-making as often as you do? Go through the list of rights you have identified as being threatened. Think about your expectations long and hard. Write this down too.

Did you agree with your partner explicitly that this was something you could expect from the relationship? Did *you* expect you would get this from your relationship, but never talk it through? Does your partner know you expect this? Does he agree?

In the long run, is this a rational thing to expect of your partner, or not? It's fine to be irrational, but you'll get further if you can recognize when you are being so.

Afterwards

Once you have thought about your rights, consider what to do next.

- If you realize that some of your expectations have actually not been discussed with your partner, then do this. It could be that he doesn't realize he is infringing your rights as you see them. It could be that you need to talk through what they are.
- Are you sure that your partner is breaking an agreement, or denying you your rights? It could be that he doesn't agree with you, and that you need to redefine what your rights are, or find a relationship where both partners agree—for example, on a common policy of fidelity.
- Is the person or thing you are jealous of *really* taking away the things you think they are? If they didn't have a place in your partner's life, would your partnership be improved? How does having this thing or person in his life make your partner more attractive (would you really love him more if he never spoke to his mother again?) What would you miss out on that your partner wouldn't be able to give you?
- Is it really in your long-term interests for your partner to give you what you are expecting? Demanding a partner's presence twenty-four hours a day, for example, may be counter-productive in the end.
- Have you identified any expectations that *you* feel are irrational? This is the time to ask for support and reassurance. You may not want your partner to change what he is doing—but you may need to reaffirm your love for each other.

Who or what am I jealous of?

What is this person (job, hobby) taking away that should really be mine?

1

2

3

4

5

What really are my rights in this situation?

Exploration 31 — Motivating each other

One of the main advantages of being together as a couple is that you can help each other to achieve things—even things you may not have much energy for. One of the gifts you can give each other is to learn just how to motivate the other—to work, to play, to empty the rubbish bin, or to take a well-earned break.

Most of us have learned the (incorrect) lesson that to motivate someone means to nag them or hassle them. It doesn't, but what is the right way to motivate each other without being manipulative? The answer is to find out the ways in which your partner naturally motivates himself, and then encourage him to use these to do something he hasn't much energy for.

The exploration

This exploration gives you both the chance to find out how your partner naturally motivates him- or herself. It takes you through the natural sequence most people use when they are keen to achieve something, and asks questions to find out how your partner does this.

First, think about something your partner really enjoys and is keen to do. It could be a sport, some work activity, or something you do together. Imagine what it is like to be your partner enjoying this and being motivated to do it. If your partner is willing, you can ask him to help you with some details. What good things does he get out of doing what he is naturally motivated to do? Then write down as many 'pay offs' as you can think of, in answer to the first exploration question in the space provided opposite. Does he play for company, the knowledge that he's getting fit, or the buzz of winning? Which is most important for him? You can use this knowledge to help your partner do something he wants to do but can't find the motivation for, like going on holiday.

What good things could he get out of going on holiday that are as similar as possible to the ones he gets out of something he already enjoys, like squash? If your partner is motivated to play squash by being with friends, perhaps a good holiday would be one where he gets a chance to socialize. If it's the knowledge he's getting fit, then how about a holiday that includes sport—like a skiing holiday, or sailing in the Greek islands?

Afterwards

The effect of this exploration only begins when you use it to motivate your partner. The questions give you information; then you have to begin to use it, to give your partner the motivation they need.

Persuade your partner not by telling him he'll feel bad if he *doesn't* do something, but that he'll feel good when he *does*. You may need to change your way of approaching the issue, but in the long run, it will have better results.

It works two ways of course. How would it be if, instead of nagging you to do something, your partner knew exactly how to make it attractive to you by telling you of all the pay-offs? Try telling him what motivates you and see what happens.

Think of something your partner enjoys and is keen to do.
What are the pay-offs of doing this thing?

Think of something your partner really wants to do but hasn't actually got around to doing. What would be the pay-offs of doing this thing that are similar to the ones that motivate him naturally?

Exploration 32 — In love forever

To build a working partnership, you need to meet each other's needs on many levels, both practical and emotional. However, we are brought up to expect more than just a working partnership. We expect love. The subject of love is a complex one, but there is one factor that seems to be present in almost everyone's experience of it. This is a feeling that with this man or woman, anything is possible. Many of us have felt this emotion, but very few of us know how to maintain it beyond the 'first flush' of a relationship.

We have talked to many couples, but we have never come across any who have maintained that feeling constantly for 40 years. However we *have* found a way to regain the feeling once it has been lost. A word of warning though: this exploration won't work unless you put yourself into it completely. If that isn't possible for you, do another exploration now and leave this one for another time.

The exploration

Begin by finding a safe place and a safe time, when you are feeling good about each other and about your relationship. It is probably better to choose a time when both of you are feeling undistracted, by work or other people, even by alcohol, a time when you are both totally there for each other and have time to talk and hug. Think about what you want out of life. In particular, think about things you want to have or to do in the future—in about 20 years' time. Then take one half of the page each, and write down on it these things:

- Four things you want and expect to get.
- Four things you want but are afraid you won't get.
- Four things you want that seem impossible. (All these things for about 20 years in the future.)

Take your time and don't be limited by thinking that anything you want is impossible. For this once, allow yourself to want anything, no matter how wonderful. When you have both finished, sit comfortably and so that one of you can (mostly) listen and the other can (mostly) talk. The one who is talking should ask their partner, in these words, for the first thing on your list:

'In the distant future, can we . . .'

The one who is listening should simply say 'yes'. This is not a promise; it is not your responsibility to give your partner what they are asking for. You are simply saying that you are aware that they really want this thing, and that you are confirming their right to have the things they want in life. You are affirming their vision. You don't need to say any other words than just 'yes'.

If you are asking, then listen to your partner saying 'yes' to you. Imagine a future together where you are working towards what you want. When you have asked for all 12 things, change over. Now it is your turn to listen, and your partner's turn to ask.

Afterwards

Remember throughout that if you are asking, you can ask for anything. If you are responding, you do not need to be sure this thing will happen—only that, for the moment, you are telling your partner that you love him and are happy to add your energy to his in getting what he wants.

Partner 1

In the future can we . . .

1
2
3
4

1
2
3
4

1
2
3
4

Partner 2

In the future can we . . .

1
2
3
4

1
2
3
4

1
2
3
4

Sex

In our society, the difference between a friend and a partner is very often defined by whether you share sex or not. It doesn't have to be this way. We have worked with happy couples who have not slept together in ten years, and we have known people who had sex with each other without ever thinking of themselves as partners. Nevertheless, sex is an important factor for partners—even if its importance lies in the fact that you have chosen not to include it in your relationship.

Sex can be seen as something special—certainly at the start of a relationship it can have a magic all of its own, as you combine learning, sharing and giving pleasure in one glorious experience. But in many ways it is like all other partner activities—it demands good communication; it can need careful negotiation; it can lead to problems when you need and want different things.

The basic skills you need are those that we recommended throughout the book. Find out what you *really* want; find out what your partner really wants; make sure you know your implicit as well as your explicit contract; and be willing to negotiate.

What are we aiming for?

It can seem that a perfect sex life must be all about what happens physically—the techniques used, the sensations explored. This is only half the story. Good sex does result in physical pleasure, but it is also about setting that pleasure in a framework of emotional satisfaction. So when we think of 'ideal' sex, we may be talking about sex that is affectionate, guilt-free and linked with careful decisions about whether it will lead to making a family as well as making love. Also, when we talk about 'ideal' sex we are talking about an aim that will change from couple to couple, and even from one time of love-making to the next. There is no ideal, just what you, as a partnership, want and enjoy.

What are we aiming for in exploring our sexuality in order to enhance it? Some of the answers we've received from couples are as follows:

'Love-making that is in the here and now'; 'Being able to say what I want and hear what he wants'; 'Knowing that we are having safe sex'; 'Always developing and changing what we do and never lapsing into routine'; 'The security of knowing that it will always be like this'; 'I need to know we are faithful to each other'; 'Knowing I'm not trapped'; 'Feeling safe and being able to explore'; 'Knowing we love each other.'

Some of these aims may be true for you, some may not mean anything. You'll notice that we don't include crises; very often for those you need specific help, not the general improvement that these pages suggest. If you don't make love any more (and are unhappy about this), if you are feeling sexually oppressed by your partner, if you have serious worries around family planning, then this may be the time to seek personal counselling (see the list at the end of the book).

High risk, low risk

Sharing thoughts and feelings about sex can be threatening. It is very easy to see a partner's desires as a statement that they are not satisfied with the status quo. However, the fact that you both care enough to change is a proof of love, not the death of desire.

It is important to set up situations where you can share your fears, hopes, embarrassments and worries with each other with particular care. We suggest that you choose your time and place for these explorations carefully; avoid times when you may get interrupted by phone, pet or child; avoid places where it's just not possible to cuddle, touch or feel strong emotion. Also, be prepared for strong emotion. Sexuality is wonderful, but often our past experiences of it have made us vulnerable and defensive. Often we do not fulfil our potential in bed because we are frightened and wary. Coming out of our protective shell and sharing such fears is a step that needs handling with care.

The explorations

What issues affect love-making? We have chosen ones that come up again and again with the couples we meet and work with.

- **Voices from the past** Firstly, we look at where you get your ideas about sex from. What past messages do you carry with you to your love-making? These can deeply affect the here-and-now of sex, as you remember the past rather than getting involved in the present. How can you choose which messages to keep and which to leave behind?

Particularly in bed when the emphasisis is on sensation rather than verbalization, it can be difficult to communicate what you really want and like. It can also be difficult to listen to your partner's preferences. These three explorations are high-risk, but are a certain way of learning more about your partnership in your most intimate moments.

- **First moves** The first exploration examines who makes the first move, and what that means for your partnership.
- **There, please** The second gives you a chance to share with each other just where your sensitive areas are, and how you like your partner to touch you.
- **Patterns of love-making** We look at patterns of love-making, how they differ and how you can exchange preferences and learn from each other.
- **Open or closed?** Next, we explore the issues around open and closed relationships. Is yours a relationship that allows for other sexual liaisons? It is worth checking once in a while that what you both agree to what it is what you both really want.
- **Contraception** Whether or not you already have a family, the issue of conception is deep-rooted and inextricably bound up with sex. It is important to be clear about how this decision will be implemented; hence an exploration on methods of contraception.

What next?

When you have done these explorations, what next? Congratulate yourselves, for you have, by discussing and exploring such sensitive issues, broken one of the great taboos of our society. To exchange information about sexual matters is unusual, even in our 'free' society. To do so in a way that will enhance a relationship is even more rare. It could be that knowing this, you will be able to discuss other matters in your relationship with more confidence and less fear. You will certainly know that your relationship is built on trust, for it takes a great deal of trust to embark on some of the explorations we suggest in this chapter.

Exploration 33

Voices from the past

When you go to bed with your partner, there may not be just the two of you there! It could be that, along with your lover, you are including all kinds of other people—or rather, their opinions and beliefs about sexuality.

Our thoughts and emotions, and the actions and reactions that come from them, are to a large extent based on our past and what we have learned from it. We learn, not only from what other people say but also from what they do, from opinions we hear, from books, films and stories we are exposed to. When we do anything, even make love, we carry with us a chorus of voices from the past.

This exploration enables you to identify what past messages you are carrying with you. Some will be useful, others you may decide you want to do without. But if you don't know what they are, you cannot begin to decide.

The exploration

The drawing contains people who may have been significant in your past. There are some gaps, in which you can put any other significant people from your life. Then, in the speech bubbles, write in the messages they have given you about sexuality and lovemaking. Did your best friend's pregnancy carry the unspoken message that sex leads to heartache? Did your parents warn you not to do it before you were married? For each person, identify one key message.

Afterwards

When you have finished, look at the messages you have. You may find they contradict each other. Some may now be unimportant to you, but many may still influence your behaviour and emotions. How? Which of your pleasures and which of your hang-ups today find their foundation in something you learned from someone else many years ago?

Remember that every person in your life has their own set of experiences about sexuality, which influenced what they told you. They may not have had a happy time in their sex life, and may have inadvertently passed their discontentment on to you. Negative messages about sex are not objective truth, just someone's bad experience—and you don't need to take that on board.

Decide which of your messages from the past you want to carry on listening to, and which you'd rather hand back to the person you got them from. Next time you find yourself feeling guilty, and realize that this was because your mother warned you never to make love with the light on, tell yourself that you are not your mother, and need not take her message on board.

There may be lots of positive messages, ones which have made your sex life delightful and positive. Be aware of them—and thank the people who handed those gifts on to you.

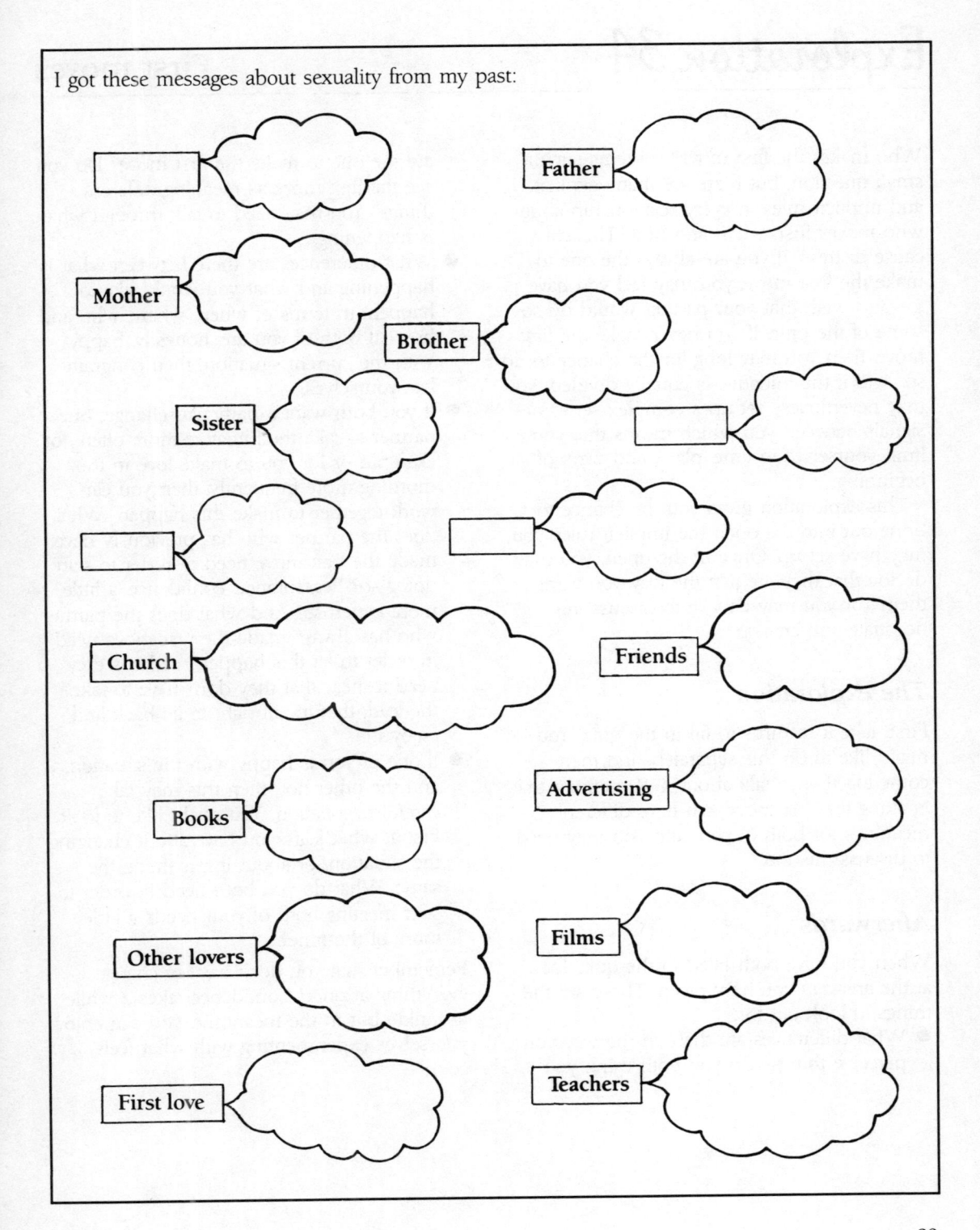

I got these messages about sexuality from my past:

- Mother
- Sister
- Church
- Books
- Other lovers
- First love
- Father
- Brother
- Friends
- Advertising
- Films
- Teachers

Exploration 34

First moves

Who makes the first move? It seems such a small question, but there are many explicit and implicit rules in every relationship about who moves first, when and how. This can cause distress. If you are always the one to make the first move, you may feel you have to—and wish that your partner would do so some of the time. If you never make the first move, then you may long for the chance to do so. And if the initiative is equally divided, you may nevertheless set up a complex series of signals between you which means that you limit yourselves to time, place, and ways of beginning.

This exploration gives you the chance to bring out into the open the implicit rules you may have set up. Once in the open, you may decide that they are just the way you want them—or you may choose to discuss, re-negotiate and change.

The exploration

First, take it in turns to fill in the quiz. You might like to do this separately and then come together to talk about it. Remember that 'making the first move' can have different meanings for both of you, and you may need to discuss this too.

Afterwards

When you have both filled in the quiz, look at the answers you have given. These are the things to look out for:
- What differences are there in the way you perceive things? Do you both think you are the one to make the first move? Do you see the first move as meaning different things? You may need to talk through what is happening.
- What differences are there between what is happening and what you would like to happen, in terms of when, where, who and how? If both of you are, honestly, happy with the current situation, then congratulate yourselves.
- If you both want a particular change; one partner to take the initiative more often, for example, or for you to make love in the morning more frequently, then you can work together to make this happen. What does the partner who has previously never made the first move need in order to start doing so? Reassurance, confidence, a little more expertise? And what does the partner who has always made the first move need in order to let this happen? Perhaps they need to hear that they don't have to take the lead, that it's all right to lie back and enjoy it!
- If one of you is happy with the situation, and the other not, then this may take careful negotiation. You might like to look first at what fears you have about changing the situation, or about it remaining the same. What do you both need in order to start meeting both of your needs a little more of the time?

Remember that you don't have to change everything at once. Confidence takes a while to build—but in the meantime, you can enjoy yourselves experimenting with what feels good!

HIM
Who makes the first move most of the time?

What percentage of the time?
How?

0% ▬▬▬▬▬▬ 100%

What percentage of the time does the other one make the first move? How?

0% ▬▬▬▬▬▬ 100%

What percentage of the time does it 'just happen'? How?

0% ▬▬▬▬▬▬ 100%

What would you like to happen that is different from the above?

HER
Who makes the first move most of the time?

What percentage of the time?
How?

0% ▬▬▬▬▬▬ 100%

What percentage of the time does other one make the first move? How?

0% ▬▬▬▬▬▬ 100%

What percentage of the time does it 'just happen'? How?

0% ▬▬▬▬▬▬ 100%

What would you like to happen that is different from the above?

Exploration 35

There, please

Making love can be totally spontaneous, a wonderful exploring of each other's bodies. But sometimes, there is a time and a place for a little more knowledge and forethought, an opportunity to tell each other just what you like without worrying whether you will spoil the heat of the moment.

The exploration

The exploration speaks for itself. Fill in on the relevant drawing your erogenous zones, and the zones you don't like touched. Then fill in what you like to your partner to do. Do it separately from your partner, or together, then swap notes. In bed, with some good food and drink, this can turn from a theoretical exploration into the nicest form of practical exercise!

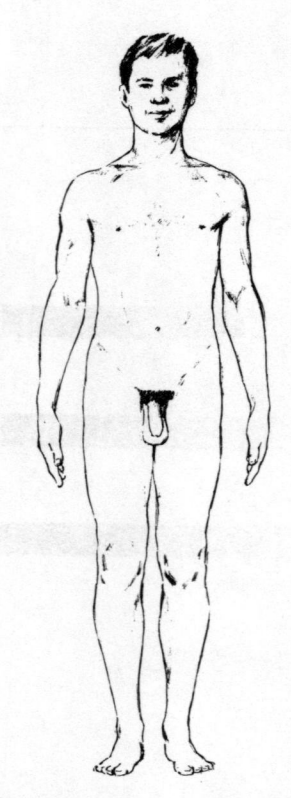

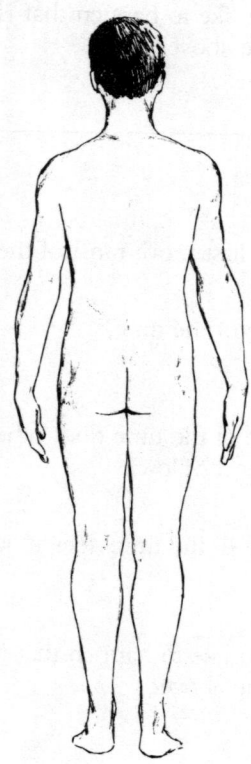

Shade in the drawing to show
   very erogenous zones
   erogeneous zones
   don't bother zones
   keep off! zones

Now show where you like to be:
   kissed
   licked
   tickled
   stroked
   . . . and invent your own of course

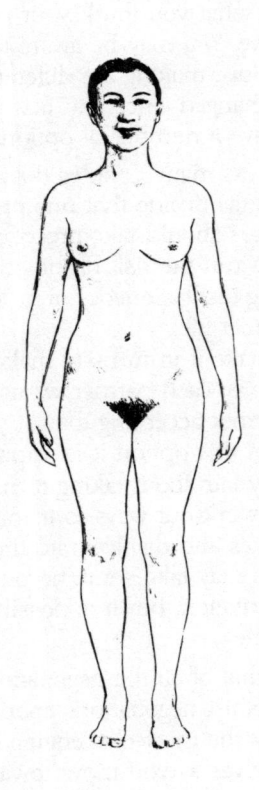

Shade in the drawing to show
   very erogeneous zones
   erogeneous zones
   don't bother zones
   keep off! zones

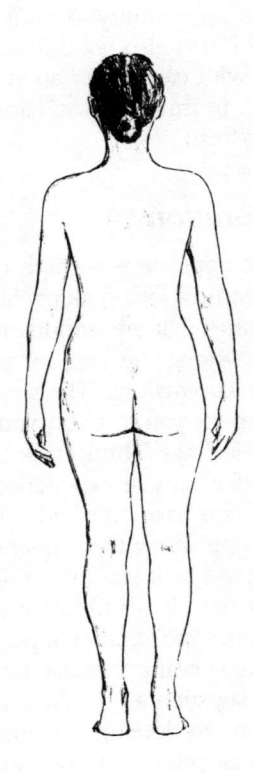

Now show where you like to be:
   kissed
   licked
   tickled
   stroked
   . . . invent your own of course.

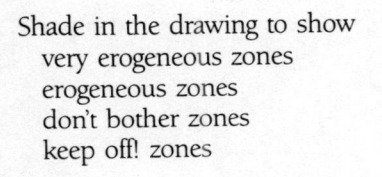

Exploration 36

Patterns of love-making

Each act of love follows a pattern. For many people, that is a slow build-up of arousal, followed by a climax, followed by a period of warm cuddling. It doesn't need to be; everyone is different, and what you need at different times is different too.

It is good to be aware of what your needs are in bed, and the ways in which they can change and develop. This exploration helps you to become more aware of your needs, gives you an opportunity to think about and explore them. It is also good to keep communicating with each other about what you need in bed. In this way, you can keep your love-making fresh.

The exploration

On the page opposite is a graph of one person's pattern of love-making. She has drawn in things that are important to her, and indicated how long she likes to spend on each part of love-making. The spaces below the graph are for you to fill in your own sequence of feelings. Think back to the sequence of feeling you experienced during the best sex you have ever had. Then mark in particular points along the sequence that made it as good as it was. You might want to include orgasm, if it is important to you; rhythm changes; position changes; penetration, if this is relevant; foreplay (and what kind); afterplay such as cuddling and talking. Take your time to develop and mark down as many things as you can, to build up a clear and detailed picture of your pattern.

Afterwards

When you have both filled in your patterns, you may want to share these with each other. Swapping papers may be one way—and another is to demonstrate just what you have realized you need, in detail! It can be enlightening to offer your partner just what they need, rather than what you thought they needed—and to accept just what you want, rather than what you think your partner wants to give. You may be aware too that your patterns of love-making are different, or that they have changed since you first met. In this case you have a number of options:

- You can (as many couples do without admitting it) decide that one partner's preferences should take precedence all the time. You run the risk of the other partner becoming disillusioned, but at least you have a quiet life!
- You can take it in turns to make love in just the way each partner wants, with the other partner accepting that; if you do decide on this option it is important to be rigorously fair about taking turns.
- You can work out ways to incorporate both sets of likes and dislikes into the one act of love. This may take some negotiation and experimentation, but it is possible and worthwhile.

Remember that of all the negotiations possible in a relationship, negotiations about sexuality are probably the most challenging. So congratulate yourselves as you move towards meeting your needs more fully.

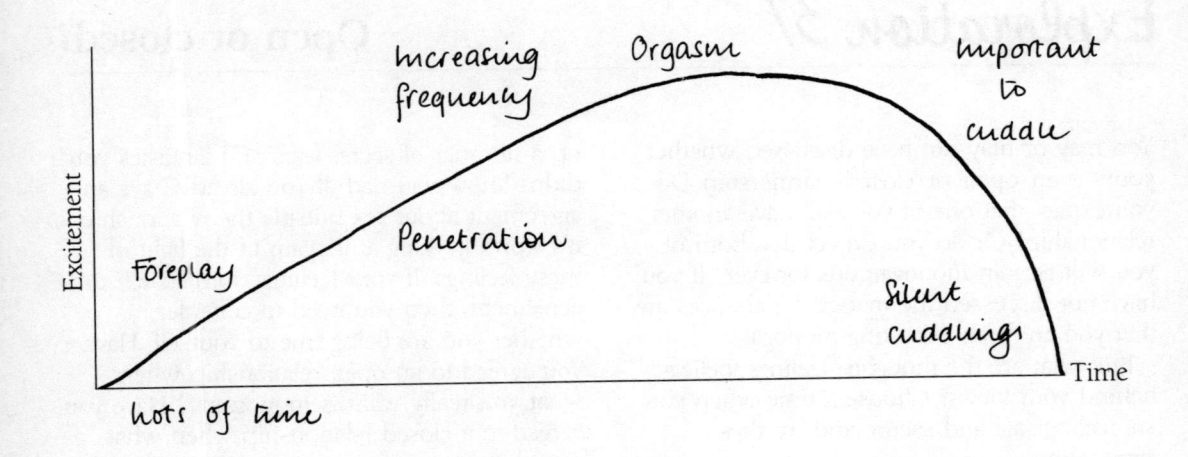

Excitement | Foreplay — Penetration — Increasing frequency — Orgasm — Silent cuddlings — Important to cuddle — Time

lots of time

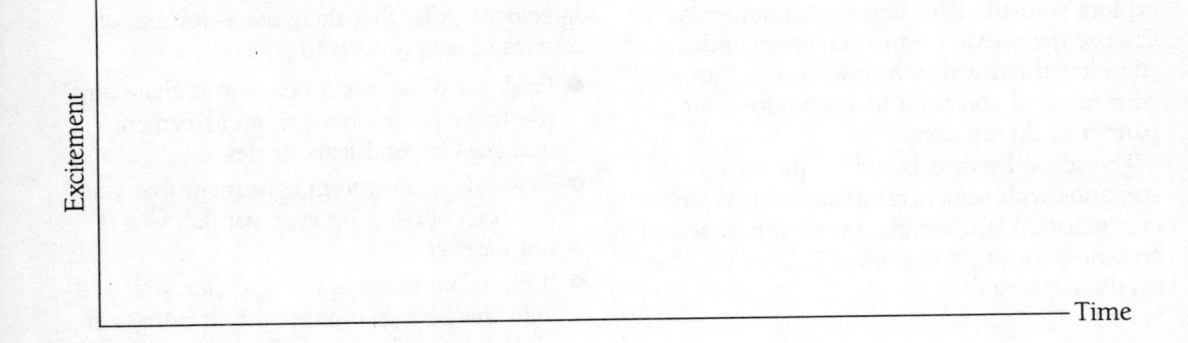

Excitement | Time

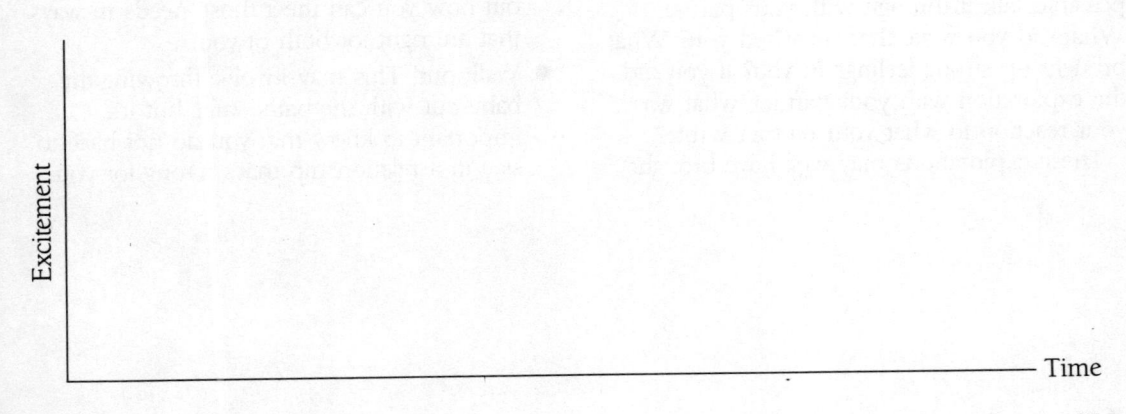

Excitement | Time

95

Exploration 37

Open or closed?

You may or may not have discussed whether yours is an 'open' or 'closed' partnership. Do you expect that one of you will have another relationship? Or do you expect that both of you will remain monogamous for ever? If you have not discussed the matter, the chances are that you are both expecting monogamy.

But what are the thoughts, feelings, beliefs behind your views? Choose a time when you are feeling safe and secure and try these explorations.

The exploration

This exploration is in two parts. It invites you explore your thoughts about your situation. Choose the relevant set of sentences and complete them with whatever comes into your mind. If you want to, encourage your partner to do the same.

The second part is based on the two scenarios with sentences about each. Whichever situation you are in, complete *both* sets of sentences. Again, it is good if both of you can do the exploration.

Afterwards

When you have completed both exercises, think about what you have written and, if possible, talk it through with your partner. What did you write that surprised you? What brought up strong feelings in you? If you did the exploration with your partner, what was your reaction to what your partner wrote?

These explorations may well have brought up a number of secret fears and fantasies you didn't know you had. If you already have an agreement about sex outside the relationship, it's worth looking at it again in the light of these feelings. If your feelings don't match the agreement, then you need to consider whether you are being true to yourself. Have you agreed to an open relationship when what you really want is monogamy? Have you agreed to a closed relationship when what you wanted was more freedom? In either case, you have taken the first step towards solving the problem—which is to bring it out into the open. The next step is to look at where you share feelings in common and have a basis for agreement. After that there are a number of courses of action open to you.

- Find out what moral beliefs you share and use those for the basis of an agreement that goes beyond fears or desires.
- Negotiate a short term agreement that you can both stick to because you know it is not for ever.
- If the relationship is too open for you, deal with the feelings of insecurity it brings up by building your own self-esteem.
- If the relationship is too closed for you, work out what feelings you have—trappedness, unfulfilled desire, curiosity—and work out how you can meet those needs in ways that are right for both of you.
- Walk out! This may involve throwing the baby out with the bath water, but it's important to know that you do not have to stay in a relationship that's wrong for you.

If you have an open relationship complete these sentences.

We have an open relationship and I believe . . .

Ours is an open relationship but I wonder whether . . .

I believe in open relationships although sometimes . . .

We have an open relationship and so . . .

If you have a closed relationship, complete these sentences.

We have a closed relationship and I know that . . .

Ours is a closed relationship, but I fear that . . .

I believe in closed relationships, even though . . .

We have a closed relationship and so . . .

Scenario 1

A and B have an open relationship. B has an affair. A gets very upset.

What do you imagine A is feeling and thinking?

What do you imagine B is thinking and feeling?

What happens next?

Scenario 2

A and B have a closed relationship. B secretly has an affair. A finds out.

What do you imagine A is feeling and thinking?

What do you imagine B is thinking and feeling?

What happens next?

Exploration 38

Contraception

If you have decided not to have a family, or not to have one yet, then you need to put that plan into action. This will involve some form of contraception. Up to 30 years ago, forms of contraception were so limited that choosing which kind to use was not an issue. Now there are many more forms of contraception, and some are currently under attack. The safest forms in terms of conception risk are not necessarily the safest for long-term health. The least likely to interfere with body chemistry may well be the ones most likely to interfere with spontaneous love-making. So the decision on which form to use is not one to be taken lightly—and as a partnership you may well want to take this decision together, weighing up the risks and inconveniences.

The exploration

The grid on the page opposite lists out seven major forms of contraception, and you may want to consider others. You can do this exploration at any stage of a relationship—just because you have been using one particular form of contraception for years does not necessarily mean that one (or both) of you doesn't have reservations about it. It is a good idea to review your family planning methods regularly to make sure that you are both happy and comfortable with them.

As you fill in the grid, list out your fears, worries, hesitations about each method—and then any advantages you may see. Some methods you may not want to use at all. Fill in the grid for these methods anyway—your partner may want to consider them.

Afterwards

Once you've filled in the grid, then compare notes. If one of you has concerns about every method, then you need to go back to square one and discuss whether in fact you want to use contraception at all.

Disregard immediately any form of contraception which you both have only concerns about. Look at the ones you each favour. If there is one method that you both favour above all others, then your task is easy.

If you differ in your preferences, particularly if these preferences have changed since the last time you considered contraception, then you need to discuss it. Things to remember are:

- The partner who seems to be blocking a particular method of contraception may be doing so because they are really frightened —for their health or about an unplanned pregnancy. They may not just be being awkward!
- If you *really* can't agree, then look at what you each see contraception as doing; it may be that one of you is chiefly concerned about pregnancy, the other chiefly about spontaneous love-making. You will need to discuss this, before you can make a sensible decision about contraception that meets both your needs.
- The method of contraception you choose does not have to be forever. You can use the pill for the next year, then change to the cap for a while.

Type of contraception	Her concerns about using it	Her reasons for wanting to use it	His concerns about using it	His reasons for wanting to use it
Pill				
Mini-pill				
Cap				
Condom				
Coil				
Rhythm method				
Sterilization/ Vasectomy				
Other				

Children

We are still a society where the expected fulfilment of any heterosexual relationship is to have children.

Certainly, this is far less the case for us than even in our parents' generation. Now we can choose whether and when to have a family, and the time is probably not too far away when we can choose the gender composition of that family too.

If you are in a situation where you feel you do not want to have children, this chapter is probably less relevant to you than many of the other chapters. It may still be worthwhile browsing through the explorations, and you should certainly do the one which invites you to consider whether you are truly committed to not having a family, perhaps trying a few of the others to test out further your reactions to the possibility.

Children—a key influence

If you are planning to have children, or have already started your family, then you will already be aware of why we include a special chapter on offspring in this book. As well as being the 'natural' outcome of a relationship, they probably affect and influence a partnership more than any other single factor. Firstly, they are the only truly irreversible event that will happen in the course of your relationship. If you split up, you can always get back together. If you buy a house, you can sell it. if you emigrate, you can always return. You cannot send a baby back. Once here, a child will alter the nature of your relationship dramatically. Not only will it interrupt the natural flow of your days (and nights), the child will add another dimension to your interaction. Rather than thinking of two people, you will now have to think about three, or four, or five. This can be an amazingly liberating experience, taking you from your concentration on yourselves out to a true unselfishness. Conversely, having another person to consider may leave you less time to consider each other. This is true at the beginning and throughout childhood, when privacy is at a premium and even the most intimate discussion is likely to be interrupted by demands for drinks of water.

Children as amplifiers

One woman we spoke to described having children as like having an emotional amplifier in the house. Whatever is going on in your relationship before the child arrives is amplified by its presence. If you are close, you will become closer. If you have rows, you will have more of them. If you are drifting apart, you will probably drift apart faster. Children pick up moods, attitudes, ideas and feed them back in an uncanny manner so that you see your own relationship reflected back.

So, children will not make your relationship suddenly become more stable but make it more of what it was. You may have to work even harder on making the relationship work, because you have a family to consider, and you will almost certainly have less energy than before to do this work.

The explorations

The explorations we have included are primarily about how to integrate children into your partnership. This is *not* a book about how to raise children, or about practical child care, but the effect that a child has on your relationship may well depend on how effective you are as a parent.

As with other chapters, the issues we look at are primarily centred around finding out each other's expectations and ideas—this time about children. With a basis of understanding between you, you will be more able to cope.

- **Shall we have children?** The first and most vital question to ask is whether to have a family at all. It is important to talk through at length all your hopes, doubts and fears about this issue in order to come to a congruent agreement. It is also important to imagine both possibilities—having children and not having them—before you finally decide.
- **What might you feel?** The most unexpected side-effect of having a family for many couples is the amount of emotion they feel about this new and very welcome person. This exploration looks at some of the range of emotions you can feel about your children, some positive and some less acceptable, and helps you prepare for this.
- **Getting support** This, the most practical exploration in the book, invites you to look at the sort of support you will need in raising your family. What needs will you (or do you) have, and how can you fulfil them in a number of ways? What will this cost you, in terms of time, money or reciprocal help? If you can, between you, agree your needs, then you will have a better chance of fulfilling them.
- **Whose responsibility?** There are many areas of responsibility in child raising, some practical, some emotional. We invite you to work out who is responsible for each area. If you are planning to have a family, this exploration will allow you to discover what each other's expectations are. If you already have a family, it is a chance to check out whether you are happy with the existing division of responsibility.
- **Giving the same message** In many of the areas of child-raising, it is vital that parents have some general agreement about the values and messages they pass on to their children. This exploration offers you a format within which to work towards some agreement in your child-rearing practice.
- **Transition points** As children grow and change, their relationship with their parents also changes. Here we ask you to look at how you can foster the right relationship with your child(ren) in order to meet their needs as well as your own, at different stages in their upbringing.
- **When they've gone** When children leave home, they gain a degree of independence. But what about the parents left behind? Alone together for the first time in many years, you will need to rediscover your relationship with each other and prepare for the remaining years without a family. This is a chance to plan for the revitalizing of your relationship.

What next?

The next step after this chapter may well be to have a family, or to work to improve the family life you already have. The main aim of the chapter, however, is primarily to help you learn more about your relationship.

It is, in fact, often within the context of raising children that couples begin to both learn more about each other and develop their relationship to its full potential. With the experience not only of birth but also of working together to bring new people into the world, many relationships find a new meaning and a new strength.

Exploration 39 — Shall we have children?

In our grandparents', or even our parents' day, the question of whether to have children was not one that was asked, because they had no choice: if you made love, you ran the risk of conceiving; if you conceived, you had the baby. Now we have a choice, which means we have the right and the responsibility to choose. It may be that the issue of whether to have children is not a matter of choice for you—either through an inability to conceive, or because your ethical viewpoint forbids contraception. But for most of us, the decision is ours: whether, when and how many children to have.

Most couples assume that they will have a family. Some assume it without talking it through, and this can be dangerous. This exploration gives you a chance to explore the options. It is best done with your partner, so that you can talk through issues together from the start.

The exploration

Imagine, first of all, a life without children. (If the decision you need to explore is whether to have more children, then imagine life with the family you already have.) Think through the future carefully, imagining what life will be like. Then answer the questions, noticing as you do so what your emotional response to each question is. It could be that answering these questions brings up problems that you need to resolve with your partner. Do this as you go, so that the answers you are left with are a full representation of what life will really be like.

Then imagine a life with children (or with more children if this is your issue). Once more, think it through carefully, imagining fully what it will be like and then answering the questions again. Once you have worked through these questions, you may well find you have a lot more information than you had when you began. Most of the problems couples have when they start a family are due to not really knowing what it will involve.

Afterwards

Pay particular attention to the questions and answers that made you react most strongly. They will usually be linked to issues you need to resolve before making a final decision. It could be that there are things you need to do before you make a final decision—making sure you have enough financial resources, moving to a house with a garden, taking that round-the-world trip. It could be that you need more information, or just time to think.

The most difficult situation is when each partner is certain of their decision—and the decisions are different. If one of you wants a family and the other doesn't, you need to think very carefully —for the child's sake if not for your own—before you act. It could be that the bottom line for one of you is that your partner's ideal future is not yours. And you may decide that you need to find someone with the same future plans as you have—be that a life of childless bliss or a family of five. Also remember that people's ideas and values change, and that waiting a while, until your relationship is more stable or your partner has clearer ideas of what he wants, may resolve the issue.

If you imagine a life without children . . .

What is the best thing about it? No responsibility

What is the worst thing about it? Cannot see personalities develop & grow. Cannot attempt most difficult life work.

What practical problems might you suffer? Feel left out of peer group.

What practical advantages might you gain? Freedom as individual / couple.

Who will approve?

Who will disapprove? Families probably.

What statement will you be making to the world? Either do not want or cannot have children.

If you imagine a life with children . . .

What is the best thing about it? opposite of worst thing above

What is the worst thing about it? 24 hr a day 365 days a year job

What practical problems might you suffer? travelling more difficult, time not your own.

What practical advantages might you gain? have fun as a family — more inclusion.

Who will approve? families.

Who will disapprove?

What statement will you be making to the world? couple who love each other & children.

Exploration 40 — What might you feel?

Becoming a parent involves many changes, some expected, some not. If you are not yet a parent, you will probably be surprised by the strength of emotion you will feel. New mothers talk with amazement about the elation of seeing and holding their own baby, but also about the depths of despair to which they can sink in the small hours of the morning when that same baby has cried all night and can't be consoled. New fathers talk about the pride of seeing this human being that they have half created, and also about the rage of resentment that can come upon them when they find themselves replaced in their partner's affections—even to the extent that she no longer wants sex.

In general it seems that the surprising thing is the strength of emotion, not the type. So if you are prone to guilt, your baby will trigger *incredible* guilt in you. If you tend to feel that you are responsible for things, the weight of responsibility for your baby will almost crush you. One woman we interviewed spoke of her despair with her child as being as deep as that of a recent bereavement. Another compared the first slap she gave her child with the guilty feelings of her first sexual encounter. A young father talked about euphoria of a kind he had only previously experienced under the influence of drugs.

The exploration

(*Do not do this exploration alone. Make sure that someone you trust is at least in the house and knows what you are doing.*)

If you are not yet a parent, but either want or expect to be, it is worth reminding yourself in advance of just how powerfully you can feel these feelings. This process is designed to take you back over times when you have experienced emotions particularly strongly. The best way to re-experience a strong emotion is to remember an emotional incident vividly.

The circles on the opposite page contain named emotions, surrounded by questions about the incident in which you felt that emotion most strongly. In the centre of the circle write in any name you have for the incident. Then take your time to answer the questions around it. You can answer them in any order, but we recommend that you take the easiest ones first. Ignore questions that don't make sense to you (they will to someone else) and remember that what is important is what you think, not what you write. Lastly, take a few moments to step into your memory and re-experience the emotions you felt at the time, or the feelings you had about it afterwards. Complete one circle at a time, and take a break before you start another.

Whether you have just got in touch with feelings of delight or of despair, you now have some idea of what having a baby will be like.

Afterwards

If the exploration brought up strong feelings in you, give yourself lots of time to come back to the present. If possible, talk it over with someone. You can also:

- Create circles for yourself based on other emotions.
- Work out what sort of support you will need when you reach your limits, and *make sure it is there*. A help-line phone number is a good start.
- Have a note ready to put up over the cot to remind you that you chose to feel these feelings because you know you can handle them.

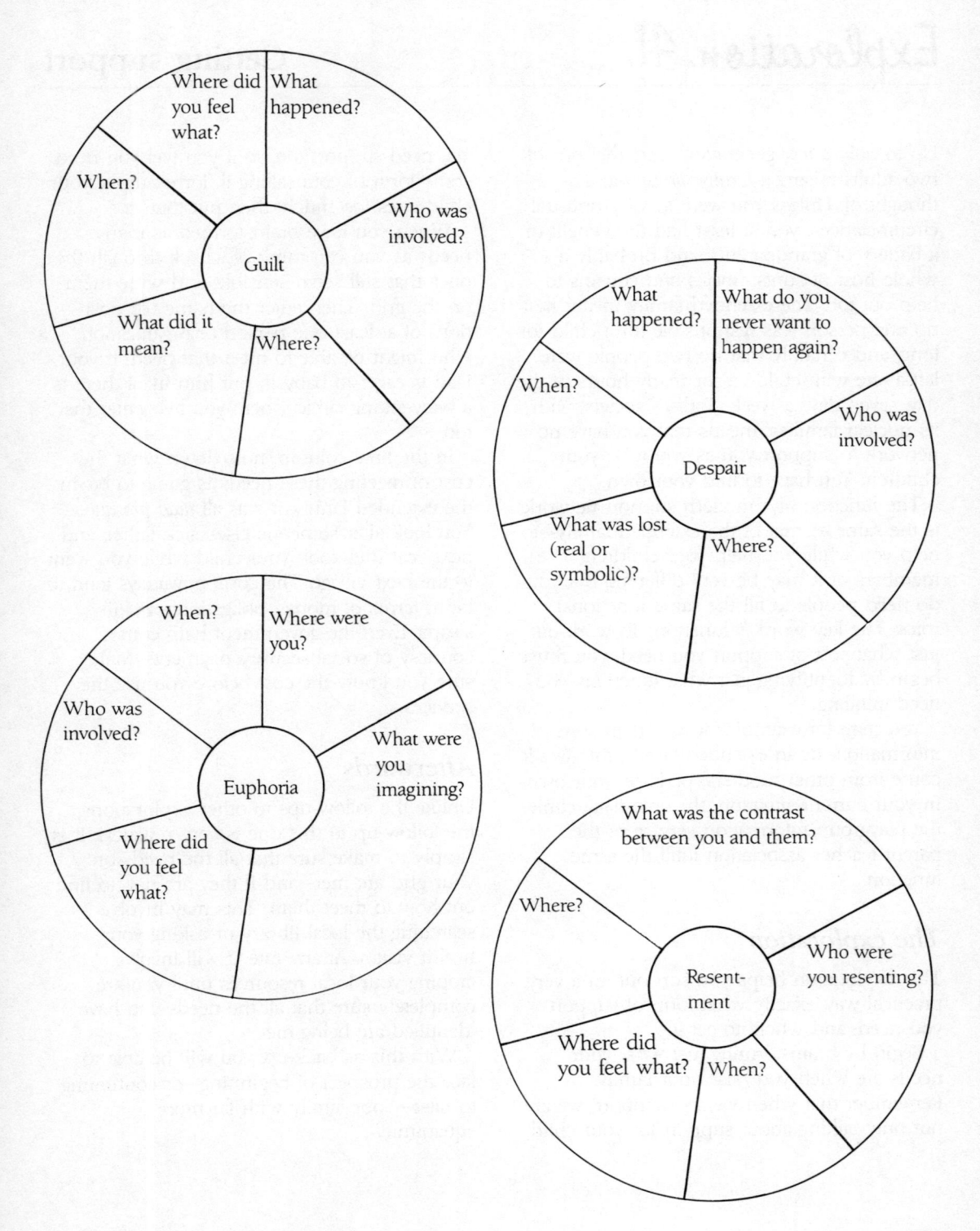

Guilt
- What happened?
- Where did you feel what?
- When?
- What did it mean?
- Where?
- Who was involved?

Despair
- What happened?
- What do you never want to happen again?
- When?
- Who was involved?
- What was lost (real or symbolic)?
- Where?

Euphoria
- Where were you?
- When?
- Who was involved?
- Where did you feel what?
- What were you imagining?

Resentment
- What was the contrast between you and them?
- Where?
- Who were you resenting?
- Where did you feel what?
- When?

Exploration 41 — Getting support

Up to only a few generations ago, the idea of two adults raising a family alone was unthought of. Unless you were in very unusual circumstances, you at least had the benefit of a battery of grandparents, and probably a whole host of aunts, uncles and cousins to help out too. The extended family meant that no one person was responsible for a child for long, and certainly that no two people were left alone with children for many hours of the day, seven days a week. Today's society, with its nuclear families, means that you have no network to support you as you raise your children. You have to find your own.

The function of a modern support network is the same as that of the extended family—to help you while you help your children. The members of it may be very different, but you do need people to fill the same functional roles. The key word is function. To work out just what sort of support you need, you must begin by identifying just what functions you need fulfilling.

You may, for example, need certain sorts of information. In an extended family, this would come from other mothers, perhaps your own. In your current situation, the ante-natal clinic, the playgroup information service or the parent teacher association fulfil the same function.

The exploration

This exploration helps you sort out, in a very practical way, exactly what form of support you need, and where to get it.

Begin by brainstorming just what your needs are when you raise your family. Remember that when we say 'support', we are not only talking about support for your child. You need support too, so if you feel you need some form of counselling if, for example, your child cries too much, then put that in.

When you have brainstormed as many needs as you can think of, check through the ones that still seem sensible, and write them on the grid. Then enter the name (or position) of at least one person or organization who might be able to meet that need. If your Dad is eager to babysit, put him in; if there is a baby-sitting circle where you live, enter that too.

In the final column, note down what the cost of meeting these needs is going to be. In the extended family, it was all *quid pro quo*. You look after someone else's sick father, and next year they took your child while you went to the next village. The costs nowadays tend to be in terms of money, obligation, or skill swaps. Even the government help comes courtesy of social security payments. Make sure you know the cost before you use the services.

Afterwards

Unlike the follow-ups to other explorations, the follow-up to this one is very practical. It is simply to make sure that all the needs on your grid are met—and if they are not, to find out how to meet them. This may involve searching the local library or asking your health visitor. At any rate, it will involve tapping your local resources until you are completely sure that all the needs you have identified are being met.

With this as back-up, you will be able to face the prospect of beginning—or continuing to raise—your family with far more equanimity.

The need	How to meet the need	The cost
Practical support Baby-sitter	Janine (Derek's sister)	£2.50 an hour
Information Library		
Emotional support Parent network		
Expertise Doctor or dentist		

Exploration 42 — Whose responsibility?

A child can seem, as she tries to climb the park railings for the fourth time, to be a totally independent being.

In fact, children depend on us all the time, for love, hugs, and vital practical support. The horrible truth is that your child is *genuinely* dependent on you for survival, and that is a heavy responsibility.

But whose responsibility is it? In theory, both parents support their children and take responsibility for their welfare. Although sometimes women do often give financial support while men do the child rearing, in practice most children are still dependent on their mother for day-to-day physical care. The feeding, bathing, changing and tucking up is still most often done by the female partner or at her instigation.

What is the situation in your partnership? Whether you are preparing for a family or coping with one already, you probably have fairly clear ideas of who will do what, how much and when. Perhaps Dad takes the children to school in the morning, but Mum collects them. Perhaps they are Mum's responsibility during the week, but at weekends it is over to Dad to cope. This creates whole areas of discussion (argument, strain, co-operation) about how you divide responsibility, and what this means for your partnership.

For example, what effect does it have if one of you has a full-time job? What happens later if the child rearing partner takes a job? Does she naturally give up some of her child rearing, or does she simply do her job on top of the prior arrangement?

The exploration

This exploration is one you can do equally well whether you have a family or are planning to have one. However, the second part of the exploration differs depending on which situation you are in.

The grid lists a variety of tasks concerned with child rearing. On one side of the page are spaces for you each to fill in your idea of who does what. If you haven't yet got a family, then these will be expectations. If you have, they will be based on reality. Take it in turns to mark in who does which job, or, if it is shared, how it is divided.

If you have no family already, then this is all you do. If you have children, go back over your marking, and tick any divisions of responsibility you are *satisfied* with. So if you have marked down that 60 per cent of the time you cook the children's meals, and 40 per cent of the time your partner does, and you are happy with this, then tick it. If you feel that this is an unsatisfactory arrangement for some reason, don't tick it.

Afterwards

- If you don't have children yet, the aim of this exploration is to sort out what your expectations are of the division of responsibility between you.

    This is vital. It probably won't stop you having a family if you suddenly discover that your partner expects you to do everything—but it should make you stop and renegotiate. It is too late to do this once the baby is there, crying for its feed.
- If you have children already, then you may not need to talk about expectations—although many couples are shocked to find they have been working for years with totally different ideas of what each is supposed to do. The real issue for you is whether you are both satisfied with the way things are, or whether you need to renegotiate.

	HER	**HIM**
Breast feeding		
Bottle feeding		
Other meals		
Changing nappy		
Bathing		
Dressing		
Washing clothes		
Ironing clothes		
Shopping for		
Looking after daytime		
Looking after evening		
Taking to playgroup/school, etc.		
Earning money to pay for		

Exploration 43 — Giving the same message

The whole issue of how to raise children is rife with conflicting ideas. What we are concerned with here is working out ways in which your ideas and your partner's do not conflict. One sure way to present a child with confusion later in life is for you and your partner to be confused about what the ground rules are now. If the two of you present an inconsistent model of the world to your child, then what she will end up with is a confused way of reacting. If Mummy says one thing and Daddy says another, a young person may well learn to play one off against the other—but she may also learn both sets of messages and both sets of values, and if the issues are deep enough, will then have trouble about which to follow—and always feel in the wrong.

The exploration

This exploration begins a process which will continue throughout the time you raise your family. It presents you with a number of topics to talk through with each other within the framework of child rearing.

The topics on the left hand side of the grid are starting points for your ideas.

Begin by jotting down under each heading your ideas as they come. You will only have room for certain key words—for example under 'socialization', you might want to write 'giving and receiving' to remind you that one of the skills you want your children to learn is that of sharing with other people. Because you are using key words in this column, you need to be sure you both know what they mean, so, once both of you have filled in your 'ideas' column, spend some time discussing what your ideas mean. Don't presume that what you mean by those words is what your partner means—putting 'must learn all the basic skills' under the heading 'education' may mean for you that your children should be literate and numerate. For your partner it may mean that they should be able to look after themselves physically.

The second column asks you to discuss your goals in raising your children. This is a deeper question. What do you want your children to be like when they are adults? What sort of upbringing would you have wanted to have when you were a child? Imagine you are your child; what sort of upbringing do you think he or she wants? Then discuss this with your partner. Notice where your goals are different, where your children may be getting different messages about what is important. As mentioned before, different messages are not necessarily a problem for children, but if the messages about key issues—such as morals, discipline, love—are conflicting, then a child will be caught. Which of the vital messages should she follow? If they are total opposites, the child will be in a position of never pleasing both parents, and so *always* being in the wrong.

The final part of this exploration then is for you and your partner to come to some general agreement about what values you present to your children. This should not be difficult, if you are a working partnership you will probably have similar values anyway, but discussing them will lead you towards an understanding and an agreement which your children will recognize.

Afterwards

This exploration needs to be done regularly, to check that as you change, you are still presenting similar—or at any rate not conflicting—messages. Working from congruence within you and between you is the best foundation for child raising.

Issue	Her ideas	Her outcomes	Agreement	His outcomes	His ideas
Discipline					
Love					
Morals					
Socialization					
Education					

Exploration 44

Transition points

Think back to your own childhood. Your earliest memories are probably of your mother, all-knowing and infinitely trustworthy. Now think about your relationships with your parents when you decided to leave home. In your late 'teens or early twenties, your understanding of your parents was far less simple.

How did this change take place? It was not a simple, continuous transition. Rather, it was a series of transitions, some small, some large. And they don't all go in the same direction. Sometimes you loved, sometimes hated, sometimes you took another step towards independence, sometimes came running back into the fold.

With your own children, you will experience these transitions from the parent's point of view. While some of these moments will delight you (Johnnie's first steps), others may be a trial (Karen coming back from the disco at 3 a.m.). In all these situations, it is important that you act in a way that really meets their needs—and yours. There are no simple rules for how to handle a transition point in a way that meets all your needs: you must rely on a combination of your own childhood experience, and on role models—particularly your own parents. The best way to prepare for this is to review all the sources of information you have now.

The exploration

The life line on the opposite page is similar to those in previous explorations, except that it runs only from birth to leaving home. On it, we have put a few transition points that your children will go through, as you did. The first step is to put in more—about ten will do. Choose points that were particularly significant to you. Here are some examples to give you ideas:

- Your first memory of being punished.
- When you realized that parents can make mistakes.
- The birth of a younger brother or sister.
- When you started to rebel.
- Battles over restrictions on boys, girls or going out late.
- Talking to a parent on an adult-to-adult basis.
- The first time you gave emotional support, rather than taking it.

Put a box around each of the transition points you have written in. In the box write in answers to whichever of these questions is relevant:

- What did you need at that time, emotionally *or* physically? Did you get it?
- What did your parents need in that situation? Did they get it?
- How have you seen other parents (or other children) deal with the same issue?

Afterwards

It may be 20 years before you use the knowledge you have just gleaned. By that time you will have forgotten the details—but you may, far more valuably, have developed the habit of both stepping back into your own childhood experience and looking to role models to become a better parent.

You can also:

- Ask friends about their childhood and adolescent transitions points.
- Talk to (and observe) other parents with children slightly older than yours.
- Take a course in parenting (check the resources section at the back for where to start).

- Leave home
- Puberty
- Start school
- Birth

Exploration 45 — When they've gone

Having children changes life. It can give you a new purpose, a new feeling of self-esteem—and it can also totally disrupt your existence. Most families survive to a greater or lesser extent; and 20 years later, the children are ready to leave, and, in theory, you can relax back into the status quo.

It is rarely as simple as that. Having a family changes you; you are no longer the young couple you were when you first met. Having a family gives you a new role, and when that disappears, you may both feel a lack of purpose, a feeling of not being valued. Also, how do you relate to each other? For so long, your interaction has been filtered through your offspring, your actions have been dictated by their needs. Now you are alone—or more alone than you have been for many years. You may have lost the art of relating.

Often, faced with a twosome where there was once a family group, couples can drift apart, or find new interests—an affair, a new partner and a new young family, an all-consuming hobby—to take the place of the ties that are no longer there.

Whether you are approaching this crisis point, or whether it is still in the far future, you can prepare for it by reviewing what resources you have to support you in this transition. You made the change from twosome to threesome; you can make it back again, with more success, because you are now older, wiser and have a relationship that has survived so much more.

The exploration

Fill in the grid together. In the first section, remember the time when you were a new couple. Recall, in detail, your goals, your problems, your delights, your ups and downs. Help each other recall the particular joy of being together, just the two of you.

Next, remember what it was like to be a family, with a new set of goals, problems, opportunities and challenges. You may still be going through this stage, or you may need reminding of various parts of it—what you learned to value about each other during the long, sleepless nights, what extra strengths you found when one of your children needed help. Remembering these things, fill in the second section.

With this knowledge, move to the third section, which asks you to put yourself into the future, a future when your family has gone. You have already made one transition successfully. How can you make this one equally well? What goals will you still have, what new joint ones can you find? What problems will you meet—how can you solve them? What new opportunities will this time in your life offer, and what new things will you find to value in each other?

Afterwards

Whether your family has left, is in the process of leaving, or is still firmly based at home, you will learn a lot about the future by filling in this grid. Think of these things:

- How will the skills you built up in making your transition from twosome to family help in making the transition back again?
- What difference do you notice in the way the two of you view the transition? If one sees it as an exciting challenge, and the other as a threat, how can you help each other to see it constructively?
- What problems can you begin planning for and overcoming now? There are many practical things you can do to offset them—moving house, taking holidays, planning joint ventures.

When we were a new couple, these were:

Our goals

Our problems (and how we solved them)

Our opportunities

The things we valued about each other

When we were raising our family, these were:

Our goals

Our problems (and how we solved them)

Our opportunities

The things we valued about each other

Now we are a couple again, these will be:

Our goals

Our problems (and how we solve them)

Our opportunities

The things we valued about each other

Futures

Does your relationship have a future? Unless you are literally ten seconds away from splitting up, then yes, of course, it does. The question is what sort of future does it have? There is a mistaken idea in our society that only relationships which last forever are valid. It's easy to think that only very longstanding couples have relationships that are worth celebrating, even if their years together have been hell on earth.

Some relationships last a few years, a few months, a few weeks—and are successful because they give both partners what they really need, and then dissolve.

It is a good idea, then, to concentrate first on the quality of any relationships you have, and to leave longevity to take care of itself. You will at least be assured of a relationship that works, even if only for a short time.

Winning futures

All that said, looking to the future in a relationship can radically improve its quality. This is one of the elements that makes commitment —be that a marriage or a ten-year mortgage together—such an attractive option. Once we can see the future with our partner, the way we see the present will often change.

Knowing that you have a future in your relationship will give you more security, more space. You can begin to trust, and to risk things—rows, confidences, sharing incomes and secrets—that are just not possible when you are always checking out whether the relationship will last. Making plans for the future, together, can make you very close. Whether that is planning a home together or a round-the-world trip, the experiences of making such plans can help you learn about each other, take each other's needs into account, and build a working partnership.

Complementary futures

A key element we found when talking to couples about their relationships was the way they saw the future. If the two of you have futures which mesh in broad terms, then you can weather the small issues, the irritations, the differences of opinion. Two people with a common vision, be it that of writing a book or having a family together, can come through crises and problems. If your future visions differ in the essentials, for example, if one of you wants children and the other doesn't, you may well find that in the ultimate analysis, you are not meant for each other. This doesn't mean that if you have deep divisions in future vision now, you will necessarily split up in the future. You may change, as often happens, so that your futures are closer together, or you may find a way of organizing your relationship so that both of you get what you want.

What kind of future?

You will each have your own ideas of what your future may be. As we have said, if you have been together for a while these may be quite similar: they will still be a result of your past, your ideals, your beliefs. To form a future that is truly right for you, there are certain ground rules:

- Think in positive terms. If you spend your time being aware of what you *don't* want out of life, it will find you. If you concentrate on what you *do* want, you will have a much better chance of getting it.
- Maintain a balance between general ideals and specifics. If you say that you want to be 'happy', then you have a general direction, but nothing specific to work towards. It may be more useful to think about how you'll know you are happy—by the fact you make love regularly, by the fact you enjoy spending time together, by the fact that you have splendid rows! Everyone's definition will vary, so be aware of what you mean by what you want.
- Are your future plans worth the time and the money you will have to put in in order to fulfil them? Check out carefully when thinking of futures that the end result will be worth it. For example, it may be that spending all that mortgage money isn't worth it, and you would much prefer to rent a flat and have more cash available for travelling.
- When you plan your futures, be aware that you need to take other people into account. If something is not right for you, you will probably have problems with it; if your actions are not right for other people, such as your partner, you will have their reactions to cope with, too.
- On the other hand, don't be swayed by other people's ideas of what your future ought to be. Your life is your life, and no one else can live it for you.

The explorations

All the explorations in this chapter look at how to identify and build the future you want.

- **The bottom line** First, we look at alternative futures with respect to your relationship. It certainly doesn't help to think about splitting up all the time, but knowing that you are not clinging to each other because you have no other choice is a positive way to view your relationship. We offer you a format in which to look at the bottom line of your partnership, and discuss it together.
- **What if?** The best laid plans can go astray when a crisis arrives. In the course of our lives, we all go through a number of crises, many of which are good, many of which are bad, all of which are totally unexpected. This exploration gives you a chance to discuss and plan, ahead of time, how you would cope. Thus you can be aware of how you and your partner may well react, and what you will need in order to cope.
- **Growing together** Every relationship is made up of interactions; some good, some bad. Couples who have grown together through the years have learned how to create positive interactions more than negative ones. This exploration helps you to learn this skill too.
- **Long term futures** This is a full-scale life-planning exercise, in which you both plan out your ideal future in terms of environment, relationship, career, family and personal development. This exploration will provide you both with a number of insights about what is important for you in your lives together, and so make it easier for you to achieve your ambitions.

What next?

The next stage beyond planning is doing. The idea of always being aware of your future and its possibilities is a good one—but in order to believe in it, you need to have proof that at least some of your dreams will come true. The next stage on from this chapter is to use what you have learned to make it happen.

Exploration 46

The bottom line

The bottom line, in any relationship, is that it comes to an end. We are not suggesting that at the first sign of trouble you should head for the door. However, unless your religion forbids it, there is always the option of leaving.

It can be that this is a good thing—not to leave, but to know that you can. If you cannot leave, then you may be stuck with a miserable existence for the rest of your life. If you *will* not leave, you may be condemning both of you to a compromise—when a future apart might have far better possibilities. Couples who choose to create better relationships apart do better for themselves—and the world they live in—than those who choose to sit it out regardless. Even if—perhaps particularly if—you know that you have a good relationship which holds the promise of lasting for the next 40 years, do consider what your bottom line is. What would have to happen for you to consider leaving? If you are clear about this, then you give yourself the added security of knowing what you want and don't want. You give your partner the added security of knowing what your breaking point is.

The exploration

The exploration asks a number of questions, and gives you each a number of spaces to fill in your answers. Remember, the more honest you are, the more you stand to gain. When you have both finished, compare your answers.

What did you discover? Is your bottom line higher than you thought, or lower? Would you leave if you knew your partner would get on better without you—or only if you thought you would get on better without him?

You may get a few shocks when you read what you have both written. Remember, your bottom line may not be the same as your partner's—or vice versa. You each have your own ways of looking at the world.

That said, many couples have found an extra security by finding out just how few things would mean a break-up.

Afterwards

You may need to talk through your answers with each other, and discuss how likely it is that any of your 'bottom lines' could happen. These are things to remember while doing so:

- There is no point in trying to reassure your partner. If you really feel that you would not go with him if he wanted to emigrate, then don't pretend you would. Your relationship is more likely to succeed if you both know what is happening.

- Writing down bottom lines will not make them happen. Just because you are talking about what it would take to split you up, does not make it any more likely to happen. If anything, knowing the score will help you both to realize just how valuable the relationship is.

HER

If any of these things happened between us, I would leave:

1
2
3

If my partner did any of these things, I would leave:

1
2
3

If I could only achieve these things by leaving, I would leave:

1
2
3

If I could see that these things would happen unless I left, I would leave:

1
2
3

HIM

If any of these things happened between us, I would leave:

1
2
3

If my partner did any of these things, I would leave:

1
2
3

If I could only achieve these things by leaving, I would leave:

1
2
3

If I could see that these things would happen unless I left, I would leave:

1
2
3

Exploration 47 — What if?

You have a good relationship. You are happy with each other, and you have financial and emotional security. If all goes well, you hope to spend the next 40 years together, and that future appeals to both of you. So what if . . .? Something is bound to happen to disrupt that vision. It might be a challenge, it might be a tragedy. One day, something will happen that will upturn all your ideas and then you will have to rethink.

This exploration is to help you lay down insurance now, in the way you think and feel about the future, to make sure that when something unexpected happens, you are able to cope with it. By exploring possible 'what ifs' you can plan what you may be able to do to cope with them.

The exploration

The exploration on the opposite page lists several 'what ifs'. Working together, add some more of your own. Then take them one by one and discuss them in depth. How would you each respond? Would each 'what if' seem a tragedy or an opportunity? How could you make the best of it, or even prepare for it now? Talk through each one thoroughly until you know not only how your partner feels and thinks about it, but that you could probably cope together.

Afterwards

The secret of doing this exploration is to learn from each other and to plan ahead. Be prepared to take practical action, if necessary far in advance, to avoid disasters and increase the possibility of euphoria.

- If a possibility is scary to both of you, then brainstorm how you could set up extra help. Would you need support from other people, from extra money, from professionals or from friends? Who could you learn from who has already coped with this and made the best of it? Who could you ask for advice?

- Do you need to do anything now in order to prepare for eventualities? It isn't a question of panicking in advance, just making sure that your fire insurance is up to date, or that you are building the sort of relationship that could cope if you did suddenly become famous!

- If it's a possibility that thrills and delights you both, why not start planning in order to make it happen!

What if . . .
we were both out of work
we won the pools
one of us were paralysed
we had triplets
the house burnt down
one of us got promoted to a job abroad
we became famous

Exploration 48 — Growing together

If you have even scanned this far through the book you will by now be familiar with the idea that you can change yourself in many different ways. But can you change your partner? Do you even have the right to want to do so? The simple fact is that you can and you do—whether you want to or not. Two people whose lives intertwine as much as those of a couple, married or otherwise, affect each other to the extent that they actually develop a joint personality. This is referred to by psychologists as the 'dynamics' of a relationship.

A dynamic is a sequence of actions between you that follows a recognizable pattern, for example the subtle dance that leads from subliminal body-language signals to lovemaking. Other dynamics lead to less pleasant conclusions—rows, for example. One of the characteristics of a dynamic is that a great deal of it is subconscious—the same phenomenon that we described as 'button pushing' in chapter 6. It is very easy not to recognize that you are pushing your partner's buttons as much as he is pushing yours, but rather to feel that he is in control and 'causing' the situation, where you are not.

By tracing the flow of a dynamic you can take control of it by changing what *you* do within it. This means that you improve both your own and your partner's happiness *and* you don't have to wait for him to initiate the change. In working within a dynamic, one place where you do need conscious collaboration is in working out what the dynamic is in the first place.

The exploration

On the opposite page there are two columns, one for an enjoyable dynamic and one for an unpleasant one. The easiest part of any dynamic to identify is the endpoint—the row, the sex or whatever—so we've put that at the top.

In each column, choose the example you want to work on and write this end point into the box. Then talk it through together, working out what you do to trigger each other's actions. You may often realize that what triggers you to a certain action or feeling is nothing more than a particular look on his face or tone in his voice, and your interpretation of that. In all probability, he'll report similar things to you. If you run out of boxes before you have reached the start-point of the dynamic, continue on a separate piece of paper. Finally, look for the point at which you can most easily change *your* behaviour, even in a small way, so as to change the rest of the sequence. Remember that while he can, and probably will, choose to change his behaviour as well, the whole secret of working with dynamics is to take action yourself rather than to sit around and wait for someone else to do it for you.

Afterwards

Obviously, the first thing to do is to make the changes you have just decided on. Here are some tips on how:

- If it's a dynamic you like, take one of the early elements and do it *more*.
- If it's a dynamic you don't like, taken an early element and do something *different*.
- Steal a bit of one dynamic, and attach it to another.
- As soon as you realize you are in an unpleasant dynamic, try skipping to the endpoint. This may sound like jumping out of the frying pan and into the fire, but in fact it often sabotages the whole process.
- When in doubt, do something—anything—you have never done before.

```
                    ┌─────────────┐
                    │    Your     │
                    │  dynamics   │
                    └─────────────┘
                   ╱               ╲
```

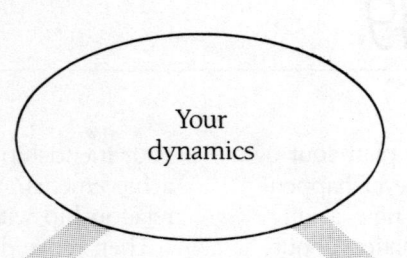

| An event we like | An event we don't like |

| The trigger | The trigger |

| What triggers the trigger | What triggers the trigger |

| What I can do to enhance it | What I can do differently to change it |

123

Exploration 49 — Long-term futures

This exploration allows you to plan your own long-term futures. They may never happen. But by fantasizing about them now, as an ideal, you gain valuable information about what you really want out of life. If you do this together, you can begin to make the ideal a reality.

The table opposite gives you four vertical columns corresponding to four key areas of your life: career, children, home, personal development. The fifth column is blank for you to add any area of your life (your religion, for example, or your love of sport) which is especially important to you. The horizontal columns begin at the top of the page with a section for 50 years from today. You may feel that you, or your relationship, will not last that long—but some of you reading this book will live for 50 more years!

Work together. Start at the top of the page and write down where you, as a couple, would ideally like to be 50 years from today. Help each other to really fantasize; no barriers as to money, talent or potential. Work across the page considering your careers first. In which direction would they go ideally? When (if ever) would you retire? How high would you rise in your career? Then consider your family. What would be your ideal child-bearing and rearing pattern? Where would your children be in 50 years? What would your relationship with them be like? What about your home; where and in what part of the world would you like to live? In what sort of dwelling? What about your personal development? What sort of person would you like to be at the end of your life? What will your friendship be like, your interests, your achievements? What will your ideal relationship with your partner be?

Then move down to the section marked for 20 years' time. What would you need to be doing in 20 years' time in order to make your dreams come true in 50 years' time? Again, encourage each other not to be limited by reality. There is far too much reality in our lives!

Move on to the section for 10 years' time. The question is the same. And so on to five years. You may find yourself becoming a little more realistic, and this is appropriate. As you move to the section for a year and a month hence, you will probably be talking about things that are quite possible for you to do.

Then fill in the very bottom section of the page with a piece of practical action that you can do right now which would be the first step on the road to your ideal. It may seem a very simple and easy thing to do (most successful first steps are) and you can give each other support to get it done.

There is no feedback or follow-up to this exploration. The thing you need to do now, to make your future lives the way you want them, is this:

- Read all the first steps for all the sections on the chart.
- Make sure that they are all things you can do easily and happily right now.
- If not, change them.
- Again, check that these are all things you can do easily and happily right now.
- Put this book down.
- Go and do them!

	Career	Children	Home	Personal Development	
Fifty years					
Twenty years					
Ten years					
Five years					
One year					
One month					
Right now					

Conclusion

Developing a relationship is a never-ending process. However successful it is, it can always be better, and you can always go to higher levels of happiness. There is no conclusion to being in love, simply a continuation.

Equally, in this book there are not loose ends for us to tie up, nothing to summarize or recap. The real content of this book is the day-to-day nuts and bolts of your particular relationship. The important part is not the explorations, but the things you find out through them. We have only provided the framework—it is up to you to supply the stuff of which this book is really composed. It is up to you to summarize, up to you to tie up your own loose ends.

Because the book is what you make of it, it doesn't end just because you reach the last page. You can go back and repeat the explorations in a month, a year, or on your golden wedding anniversary. They will still be valid, and if you tackle them with an open mind, you will still learn just as much from them. In the event of your beginning a new relationship, we also suggest you introduce this book and its ideas into the day-to-day workings of that partnership too. You could even hand it on to your children, when they get together with someone special.

Outside support

Like any book, this book has limits. There, 'on-paper' explorations stop and other support is needed. We said in our introduction that this is not a book for couples in crisis. However, you do not need a crisis to find real use in outside help to move your relationship on. If you feel you need more than this book can offer, the next logical step is to develop your relationship further with the help of another person, someone trained and expert in helping relationships reach their full potential. Use this book as a diagnostic tool to help you see when you do need outside support. Be aware of which explorations you would want someone else's viewpoint, or intervention, in dealing with.

Other indicators are these:
- Are you simply stuck, committed to each other, still in love, but aware that you are too close to each other to really help?
- Are you at a point where communication is ceasing? Is it becoming difficult even to mention your problems, let alone talk them through and resolve them? One or both of you may have built up reservations about confiding in the other.
- Is one partner using 'escape routes' to avoid dealing with real-life issues? If the only way your partner can cope with life, or with you, is to become an alcoholic, a workaholic or a junkie, then you both need expert help. Your partner cannot be expected to cope alone, and neither can you.
- Is one of you unhappy and the other not? Counselling doesn't have to be for couples. In a situation where one partner is satisfied with the status quo, it may be difficult for them to support a dissatisfied partner,

simply because they don't see what the problem is.
- Do you feel that you need an injection of new energy into your interaction? Whilst still happy with the present, and the future you have planned out, do you feel that things could be even better?

We can cope

You may have natural resistance to seeking outside support for your intimate relationship. There are several things to remember here.

In past ages, you would both have had a great deal more support from your community than you are, in all likelihood, getting now. As we point out in the introduction, you would not only have had far more first-hand experience of other people's relationships, but you might also have each had a host of same-sex relatives and friends in whom to confide, all of whom have known you since childhood. Nowadays, you often live many miles from your home town, make new friendships every few years, and limit your intimate contacts to one or two, rather than a whole village. It is no wonder, then, that 'professional friends' have had to be invented, people whose expertise is gained in formal training rather than by knowing their 'clients' from childhood. Such experts have a very real role to play, in guiding, supporting and acting as a mirror in which we can see ourselves and our relationships reflected, and so learn more about them and their development. Being aware of how your relationship can be improved does not mean that it is failing. Seeking outside support does not mean you are at the end. We see many people in the course of our professional work who have good, lasting partnerships but who want something better. To do the same, all you have to do is to go and ask.

Going to ask

There are a number of ways of getting outside support.
- Obviously, you can, as many couples do, confide in friends or relatives. Be careful, though, that they are not too close to the situation to see what is really happening. Many people tend to assume that if you confide in them about a relationship, there is a problem. If you want more happiness and what they are offering is a quick divorce route, then you may have difficulties.
- Outside agencies are often very helpful. They have the expertise and the training to help you. Most are happy to work either with individuals or couples, whether married or not. Your involvement will usually need to be in terms of a regular time commitment and sometimes, though not always, in terms of money.

You will find that working with a counsellor is like doing the explorations in this book. You will often be asked to consider challenging questions about what you think and feel. You might also be encouraged to share your feelings with your partner, to fantasize about possible futures, to think back to how your past has affected your present. You should always be left in charge of how far you go, how fast.

What now?

The quality of your relationship, and of your life, can always be improved. By the time you have worked your way through the explorations in this book, you will be either exhausted, adddicted—or both!

Exactly how you choose to explore beyond this point is up to you. We wish you luck, and hope to meet you on the trail one day.

Resources

This is a list of some of the organizations we have found useful both in building our own relationship and in writing this book.

Relate (The National Marriage Guidance Service, Herbert Gray College, Little Church Street, Rugby CV21 3AP. Tel 0788 73241) offers support counselling for individuals and couples. Look in your local telephone directory under 'Marriage Guidance'.

Association for Family Communication (44 Caversham Street, London NW5. Tel 01-485 8535) runs courses to help parents cope.

Association for Humanistic Pyschology (62 Southwark Bridge Road, London SE1 0AU. Tel 01-928 8254) is an organization for many forms of humanistic counselling and therapy and will be able to refer you to a variety of support in many disciplines.

Association for Neuro-Linguistic Programming (c/o 100b Carysfort Road, London N16) is the umbrella organization for neuro-linguistic programming, a branch of psychology upon which many of the ideas in this book are based.

British Association for Counselling (37a Sheep Street, Rugby, Warwickshire CV21 3BX Tel 0788 78328) runs counselling courses and can also refer you to counsellors in your area.

Co-counselling International (c/o Cris Nikolov, 79a Ferme Park Road, London N8 9SA) Co-counselling is a branch of self-help therapy which encourages the expression of your emotions, and has given rise to many of the ideas in this book.

City Health Centre (36-37 Featherstone Street, London EC1Y 8QX. Tel. 01-251 4429) is Ian Grove-Stephensen's London base offering individual and couple therapy.

Write to us if you have any questions or comments on any of the topics mentioned in this book. We would be pleased to hear from you via the publisher.